Assessing Common Mental Health and Addiction Issues With Free-Access Instruments

Assessment instruments are critical tools for mental health professionals. Yet, as health care costs rise, so too do the costs of these instruments, to the extent that some have become prohibitively expensive. However, the Internet offers a host of more affordable and equitable alternative assessment tools, from some of the leading names in mental health assessment instruments, and at little or no cost. The pitfall of this alternative, thus far, has been the lack of vetting and quality assessment. *Assessing Common Mental Health and Addiction Issues With Free-Access Instruments* provides the first analysis and assessment of these tools. This resource identifies the most efficient free-access instruments and provides summary information about administration, scoring, interpretation, psychometric integrity, and strengths and weaknesses. The book is organized around the most common broad-range issues encountered by helping professionals, and, whenever possible, provides a link to the instrument itself. This is an essential text for all mental health professionals looking to expand the scope and range of their assessment instruments.

Katie M. Sandberg, MA, is a national certified counselor, mobile mental health counselor, and a member of both Psi Chi, the International Honor Society in Psychology, and Chi Sigma Iota, the International Honor Society in Counseling. She has authored numerous textbook chapters, supplemental instructional materials, and a professional journal article currently undergoing publication in the fields of lifespan, and human development and assessment.

Taryn E. Richards, MEd, is a national certified counselor and a professional secondary school counselor in Maryland. She has authored textbook chapters, supplemental instructional materials, and a professional journal article currently undergoing publication in the fields of lifespan, and human development, treatment, and assessment.

Bradley T. Erford, PhD, is the 2012–2013 President of the American Counseling Association (ACA) and a professor in the school counseling program of the education specialties department in the School of Education at Loyola University, Maryland. He has authored or edited more than 15 books. He has received numerous awards for his scholarship and service to the counseling profession from ACA and the Association for Assessment in Counseling and Education (AACE).

Assessing Common Mental Health and Addiction Issues With Free-Access Instruments

Katie M. Sandberg,
Taryn E. Richards, and
Bradley T. Erford

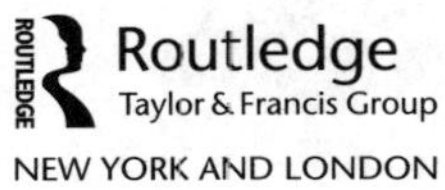

NEW YORK AND LONDON

First published 2013
by Routledge
711 Third Avenue, New York, NY 10017

Simultaneously published in the UK
by Routledge
27 Church Road, Hove, East Sussex BN3 2FA

Routledge is an imprint of the Taylor & Francis Group, an informa business

Library of Congress Cataloging in Publication Data
Sandberg, Katie M.
Assessing common mental health and addiction issues with free-access instruments/Katie M. Sandberg, Taryn E. Richards, and Bradley T. Erford.
pages cm
Includes bibliographical references and index.
1. Psychiatric rating scales. 2. Mental illness - Diagnosis.
3. Psychological tests. I. Richards, Taryn E. II. Erford, Bradley T.
III. Title
RC 473. P78526 2013
616.89'075-dc23
2012037989

ISBN: 978-0-415-81312-9 (hbk)
ISBN: 978-0-415-89829-4 (pbk)
ISBN: 978-0-203-80246-5 (ebk)

Typeset in ITC Legacy Serif
by Swales & Willis Ltd, Exeter, Devon

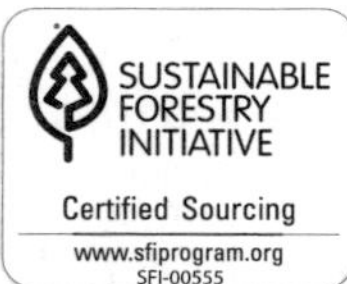

Printed and bound in the United States of America by
Walsworth Publishing Company, Marceline, MO.

This book is dedicated to my boyfriend, Rich, and my parents, Kurt and Amy, who have always believed in me and pushed me to do my best. This book would not have been possible without your patience, understanding, and support. I would also like to thank Dr. Erford for his continual faith in my abilities and exceptional mentorship.

—— Katie M. Sandberg

I dedicate this book to my loving family and friends, for their unwavering support - my anchor amidst the storms of life. I'd like to thank Dr. Bradley Erford for believing in my abilities as a writer and providing me with this opportunity.

—— Taryn E. Richards

This effort is dedicated to The One: the Giver of energy, passion, and understanding; Who makes life worth living and endeavors worth pursuing and accomplishing; the Teacher of love and forgiveness.

—— Bradley T. Erford

Contents

Chapter 3
Assessment of Mood Disorders 21

Chapter 4
Assessment of Addiction and Related Disorders 39

Chapter 5
Assessment of AD/HD, Disruptive, Impulse Control, Obsessive Compulsive and Related Disorders 57

CHAPTER 1

Introduction and Use of Free-Access Assessment Instruments

USE OF ASSESSMENT INSTRUMENTS

Along with health care in general, the costs of published assessment instruments and mental health assessment services continue to rise. However, the increasing prominence of the Internet has modified the landscape of mental health and addiction treatment services and can contribute to cost savings and higher quality services for helping professionals and their clients. Today, numerous moderate to high quality instruments are available for free use on the Internet. Unfortunately, few sources exist which systematically critique and vet the quality of these instruments. Therefore, the purpose of this book is to identify the most efficient free-access instruments, across common diagnostic categories, encountered by mental health professionals and to provide summary information about administration, scoring, interpretation, psychometric integrity, and strengths and weaknesses. It is our hope that helping professionals can use the recommended free-access instruments outlined in this book to enhance their assessment of the most commonly encountered broad range psychological issues. But first, let's cover a few basics.

What is Assessment?

Those of us who join the helping professions likely do so based on innate desires to both understand and help others. We are drawn to the challenge of furthering our understanding of human thought and behavior in order to assist others in their journey through life. The most challenging part of our profession is that the uniqueness that makes each individual so fascinating also inherently makes his or her thoughts, beliefs, attitudes, and behaviors less predictable. Already unique at birth, human beings are constantly learning, growing, and changing as a result of their individual life experiences. So how can we possibly attempt to harness what we do know about human development, behavior, and cognition in order to enhance our understanding and ultimately provide the help that many individuals seek?

This is where assessment comes in. Although no clinician can ever expect to know everything about a client or be able to predict the client's actions with perfect accuracy, assessment can help the clinician to narrow that which is unknown. Effective assessment can thus be likened to putting on a pair of eyeglasses, because it enables the clinician to sharpen his understanding of the client, focus more successfully on the most relevant clinical information, and gain confidence in his conclusions. Thus, using the best available assessment instruments can help clinicians gain clarity, focus, and confidence – all without the headache that comes from guessing one's way through blurry and unknown territories without some expert help.

More specifically, assessment is defined as the systematic gathering and documenting of client information. This can include information about the individual's knowledge, skills, attitudes, beliefs, and behaviors. Clinicians begin the assessment process the moment they meet their potential clients. From this point forward, clinicians continue to gather data, refine impressions, plan treatments, and evaluate treatment outcomes. At times, the assessment process is more formal or structured than at other times, but professional counselors are continually gathering information to aid in their understanding of their clients. It is imperative that practicing counselors use the best assessment tools at their disposal in order to efficiently and effectively help their clients.

The terms *assessment* and *test* are often, mistakenly, used synonymously. Assessments involve a systematic gathering of client information from multiple sources, while tests provide only one source of information about a client. Thus, assessments are distinguished from tests or instruments because testing is only one part of the assessment process. Tests yield important data about clients, but clinicians must use multiple sources of data and their own perceptions and judgments to make broad assessments. The instruments included in this book are mainly classified as tests. It is the responsibility of the professional counselor to supplement any knowledge gained from these recommended instruments with additional tests, observations, and clinical judgment, in order to best understand and help clients.

Because the majority of surveys, inventories, and instruments recommended in this book are categorized as tests, it is important to further define "tests." Anastasi and Urbina (1997, p. 4) described a psychological test as "an objective and standardized measure of a sample of behavior." The word *measure* tells us that the test will help us to determine "how much" of a construct or concept the client possesses. Knowledge of "how much" intelligence, depression, substance use, or extraversion the client possesses can help the clinician to predict client behaviors and analyze strengths and weaknesses in order to enhance understanding and treatment.

A test also helps clinicians to pinpoint a *sample of behavior*. Clinicians should ensure that the sample of behavior they obtain is representative of the client's typical behavior. For example, a client may behave differently when in school, work, or home settings, or when surrounded by different individuals in his or her life. It is important that tests accurately represent as many potential domains as possible in order to assess a representative sample of behavior. Tests which provide representative samples of behavior are the most likely to yield valid scores.

Finally, instruments must be *standardized* and *objective* to be considered a psychological test. Standardization means that the test is administered, scored, and interpreted in the same way for every client. Thus, two clinicians administering the same test to the same client should obtain identical scores, because all other factors are held constant. Standardization thus ensures objectivity, such that clinician bias will not affect the client's scores. It follows that, as tests are held to progressively higher standards of standardization, objectivity of interpretation inherently increases, as well.

Overall, test developers strive to produce high quality tests which will aid in the best possible understanding and treatment planning of client problems. Ultimately, it is the responsibility of the professional counselor to select the optimal psychological tests to use as part of the assessment process. Thus, professional counselors must seek to select the best psychological tests to use with various populations based on psychometric strengths and a judicious evaluation of the test's advantages, disadvantages, and ethical considerations.

In addition, prudent test authors caution clinicians that test results should always be supplemented with additional testing and clinical judgment. Although this point will be reiterated throughout the text, it should be emphasized that using multiple sources of information to understand the client and plan treatment is always the best course of action.

Purposes of Assessment

There are four main purposes of assessment: (a) screening, (b) diagnosis, (c) treatment planning and goal identification, and (d) progress and outcome evaluation (Erford, 2013). The majority of the assessment instruments covered in this book are most appropriate for use in screening, treatment planning, and progress evaluation. Assessment for the purpose of diagnosis is not as well represented among these instruments, because diagnosis requires a trained professional to use multiple sources of information in combination with clinical judgment to make well-informed diagnoses. Thus, the singular psychological tests included herein do not provide adequate information for clinicians to make diagnoses, although they are certainly useful in informing preliminary predictions which clinicians can pursue further with additional assessment.

Screening

Screening instruments are used to determine whether further diagnostic assessment is necessary or warranted. Consequently, screening instruments are typically relatively brief; thus, they likely do not comprehensively cover all possible aspects of the psychological construct in question. Screening instruments are sometimes held to lower psychometric standards than diagnostic instruments. However, the accuracy of screening instruments is just as vital as the accuracy of diagnostic instruments, because accurate screening instruments can save both the client and practitioner time, money, and emotional distress.

Screening instruments usually compare an individual's test score to a fixed cut-off score to determine if additional assessment is warranted. Cut-off scores are often set so that an individual must exceed a certain threshold of symptom quantity, frequency, or intensity in order to warrant clinical attention. Alternatively, some screening instruments are based on population norms, and cut-off scores identify those individuals who score in the extreme highest or lowest percentiles (i.e. <5th percentile or >95th percentile).

Clinicians ideally want to maximize accurate decisions and minimize inaccurate decisions when using screening instruments. Accurate decisions include identifying true positives, or clients who have the condition and are identified by the screening test as having the condition, as well as true negatives, or clients who do not have the condition and are identified by the screening test as not having the condition. Inaccurate decisions, on the other hand, include identifying false positives, or clients who do not have the condition but are identified by the screening test as having it, and false negatives, or clients who do have the condition but are identified by the screening test as not having it. False positives result in a waste of time and money and can negatively affect the falsely identified client through labeling bias and emotional distress. False negatives are even more problematic than false positives, because those who actually have the condition in question are unable to access further testing which leads to diagnosis and treatment. Thus, these individuals slip through the cracks of the system and are forced to endure the problems of their conditions without clinical treatment.

Test authors and reviewers commonly report the accuracy of their screening tests by describing the instrument's sensitivity, specificity, false positive error, false negative error, and efficiency. Sensitivity refers to the instrument's ability to accurately identify true positives, while specificity refers to the instrument's ability to accurately identify true negatives.

Both sensitivity and specificity should ideally be maximized in order for a screening instrument to accurately classify the majority of cases. For example, if an anxiety instrument yields a sensitivity of .90 and a specificity of .85, this means that 90% of individuals with anxiety were correctly identified as having anxiety while 85% of individuals without anxiety were correctly identified as not having anxiety. These values also tell us that 10% of individuals who truly did have anxiety were missed by the instrument and 15% of individuals who did not have anxiety were incorrectly identified as having anxiety. Depending on the goals and preferences of the researcher or clinician, and the intended purpose of the screening instrument, these values may or may not be acceptable. For some instruments, changing the cut-off score to a more extreme or less extreme value allows the clinician to maximize either sensitivity or specificity, depending on his preferences.

In addition, false positive error and false negative error values identify the percentage of false positives and false negatives that an instrument identifies. The efficiency of an instrument can be calculated by finding the ratio of total correct decisions to total overall decisions. Overall, when accurate decisions are maximized and inaccurate decisions are minimized, the efficiency of an instrument will be high.

Many of the instruments included in this book were designed to be screening instruments. They thus provide an efficient first step in the assessment process and enable the practitioner to identify which clients need further diagnostic assessment. Habitual use of these screening instruments in practice can save the mental health practitioner a great deal of time and money. The use of screening instruments in schools, doctors' offices, and research settings is also advantageous, because individuals with less clinical training are often qualified to administer these simple, yet efficient and effective, initial assessment instruments.

DIAGNOSIS

After screening instruments have been used to identify likely diagnostic cases, the clinical practitioner must use diagnostic assessment to determine whether these clients represent true cases. Diagnostic assessment is thus a much more detailed and comprehensive analysis of an individual, often involving a battery of tests. Clinicians must undergo substantial training and spend a considerable amount of time using multiple measures in diagnostic assessment to make a more definitive classification decision.

Diagnostic assessment can be used for the sole purpose of gathering extensive information about client strengths and weaknesses to enhance normal development, such as when a client presents for career counseling or premarital counseling. But it is most often used for the purpose of classifying an individual into a diagnostic category. Most professional counselors, psychiatrists, psychologists, and social workers use the *Diagnostic and Statistical Manual of Mental Disorders—Fifth Edition* (*DSM-5*) (APA, 2013) to make such classifications, which is the equivalent of the *International Classification of Diseases* (ICD) for physicians. The *DSM-5* delineates specific, standardized, criteria which clients must meet in order to be diagnosed with various psychiatric conditions.

Clinical diagnosis with the use of the *DSM-5* is thus helpful, because it allows clinicians to enhance their understanding of the disorder in general and then apply that knowledge to select the most appropriate interventions for maximally effective treatment. However, widespread use of the *DSM-5* is not without criticism. Because society attaches a stigma to mental illness, diagnostic labels may exacerbate the stigma by enhancing the public's view of those with mental illness as different to the average individual (Corrigan, 2007). The repercussions of being a member of a stigmatized group, and the potential harmful effects of labeling, can be devastating. In addition, over-reliance on the *DSM-5* for diagnosis can cloud the clinician's ability to consider alternative explanations for abnormal behavior (Duffy, Gillig, Tureen, & Ybarra, 2002). Therefore, clinicians are urged to take the utmost care and follow standardized procedures in order to accurately diagnose their clients.

Treatment planning and goal identification

One of the most important purposes of assessment is to assist clients and counselors in goal identification and thereby inform treatment planning. Well-defined, measureable, goals are crucial for the counselor and client to evaluate progress throughout the counseling process and make any necessary adjustments or changes.

Initial assessment procedures, often composed of standardized tests and interviews, can help the counselor uncover the most notable strengths and weaknesses of the client. This individualized information is incredibly useful in planning the most effective treatment for each client. For example, one of the instruments reviewed herein, the Autism-Spectrum Quotient, assesses the extent of autistic traits in adults with normal intelligence (Baron-Cohen, Wheelwright, Skinner, Martin, & Clubley, 2001). A client's responses on this instrument could show a clinician the domains in which a client is most resourceful and those which prove more challenging. For example, a client's responses might indicate that he has poor social skills but impressive imagination. The clinician could then use knowledge of these strengths and weaknesses to set treatment goals and gain insight into those individualized treatment options which would maximize the client's strengths. Consequently, using assessment instruments to reveal key challenges and strengths of the client enables the clinician to plan the most effective treatment.

Progress and outcome evaluation

The next logical step after goal setting and treatment planning is for the counselor and client to embark upon the treatment process. In order to ensure that the treatment selected is proving helpful to the client, it is ethically and professionally imperative that the counselor evaluate the treatment process, both throughout treatment and prior to termination, to ensure that treatment has been beneficial for the client. If a counselor fails to provide periodic checks to ensure that treatment is efficacious, the client could potentially be wasting precious time and money, and, even worse, could still be suffering from the problems which brought the client to seek counseling in the first place. Assessment instruments, such as tests and inventories, provide useful information which can be objectively compared throughout the treatment process in order to measure success.

In order to chart the progress of clients, clinicians must first seek to establish a baseline measure of the client's functioning. Clinicians typically make such an evaluation during an intake interview, initial assessment, or when counseling goals are mutually agreed upon. Progress evaluation would then follow periodically throughout the counseling process. The counselor should, at various points throughout treatment, administer the same measure used to judge baseline functioning, and then compare baseline scores to present scores in order to gauge improvement. The clinician and client may even elect to consider discontinuation of treatment once a certain score has been achieved, if that score is set as a terminal goal which would indicate success.

Baseline and continuous evaluation measures are often quite formal and objective in nature. For example, a client seeking treatment for schizophrenia may be asked to complete the Psychotic Symptom Rating Scales (PSYRATS), which assesses the severity of various dimensions of auditory hallucinations and delusions (Haddock, McCarron, Tarrier, & Faragher, 1999). The detailed information about psychotic dimensions supplied by responses on the PSYRATS can enable clinicians to enhance their understanding of these symptoms in order to plan treatment and also adapt treatment according to which symptoms are responsive or resistant to treatment. Consequently, the PSYRATS is useful throughout the treatment process as a formative and summative assessment of progress in order to ensure that clients are continually receiving efficacious treatment. In addition, the measure of distress included in the PSYRATS enables the clinician to assess overall treatment outcome as a function of change in distress, as well (Steel et al., 2007).

However, progress and outcome evaluation measures can also be informal and subjective in nature. An example of an informal, subjective, assessment of treatment progress might be a practitioner asking the client to provide a rating between 1 and 10 at the beginning of each session to index progression toward goals or overall level of distress. Subjective measures are just as important as objective measures, because the client's perception of progress is critical to alleviating distress, improving symptomology, and investing in continued treatment.

In conclusion, the four purposes of screening, diagnosis, treatment planning and goal identification, and progress and outcome evaluation are all important functions of assessment in the counseling process. The instruments reviewed herein cover each of the aforementioned purposes of assessment, and some instruments even serve multiple purposes. Prior to selecting an instrument for use, it is important that clinicians consider the purpose for which the instrument was originally intended. It is not appropriate to use screening instruments for diagnosis, and instruments useful for treatment planning may or may not be appropriate for use in progress evaluation. Clinicians are therefore urged to thoroughly familiarize themselves with the intended purpose and appropriate past use of instruments before using the instruments themselves.

CONCLUSION

We hope that the reviews of free-access instruments provided in this book can assist practitioners in providing high quality services at a fraction of the cost of using published instruments. The instruments recommended in this book were selected for review after careful evaluation of instrument purpose, target audience, psychometrics, and advantages and disadvantages. As the Internet continues to expand and increasing numbers of practitioners publish new free-access instruments, and use and evaluate extant free-access instruments, the potential for the sharing of knowledge and the use of high quality instruments only stands to rise exponentially.

CHAPTER 2

Assessment of Anxiety Disorders

PRIMARY ANXIETY DISORDERS COMMONLY ENCOUNTERED IN CLINICAL PRACTICE

Anxiety disorders are among the most commonly diagnosed mental health conditions affecting children and adults (Esbjorn, Hoeyer, Dyrborg, Leth, & Kendall, 2010; McLean et al., 2010). The National Comorbidity Survey estimated lifetime prevalence rates of anxiety disorders in the United States at 28.8% (Kessler, Berglund et al., 2005; Kessler, Chiu, Demler, & Walters, 2005). With the development of the most recent edition of the *Diagnostic and Statistical Manual of Mental Disorders* (*DSM-5*; APA, 2013), many of the criteria for anxiety disorders have been modified.

The *DSM-5* recognizes the following anxiety disorders: separation anxiety, panic disorder, agoraphobia, specific phobia, social anxiety, generalized anxiety, substance induced anxiety, anxiety disorder associated with a known general medical condition, other specified anxiety, and unspecified anxiety. Several disorders have been removed from this category, including acute stress, posttraumatic stress, reactive attachment, and adjustment disorders, which are now classified as trauma and stressor related disorders (APA, 2013). Obsessive compulsive and body dysmorphic disorder are also no longer considered anxiety disorders, and are categorized as obsessive compulsive and movement related disorders. With reclassification of these disorders, some instruments may lose their relation with the *DSM-5*, as their assessment of anxiety may include items pertaining to trauma, stressor, or obsessive behaviors. The following section will give a brief overview of the diagnostic criteria according to the *DSM-5* for each disorder.

Separation anxiety disorder involves an extreme level of anxiety, which is inappropriate for an individual's developmental age, when a person is separated from his home or a person to whom he is attached (APA, 2013). Separation anxiety is not uncommon, as lifetime prevalence rates are estimated at 5.2% (Kessler, Berglund et al., 2005; Kessler, Chiu et al., 2005). Separation anxiety is only diagnosable in individuals younger than 18 years of age. Symptoms that may occur include constant worry about the death or estrangement of the attached individual; refusing to attend school, work, or other events; refusal to fall asleep due to anxiety of separation; nightmares of separation; and physical ailments such as headaches or nausea when separation is possible (APA, 2013). Any of the aforementioned symptoms must persist for several months to qualify for diagnosis, and must significantly and frequently impede social, academic, or occupational functioning.

Panic disorder is characterized by unexpected and repeated panic attacks over time (APA, 2013). It is diagnosable if the attacks are followed by at least one month of constant fear of another attack or change of daily routine to avoid a possible attack. The panic attacks must also occur without the presence of a substance, medical condition, or mental disorder. Lifetime prevalence estimates for this disorder in adults is 4.7% (Kessler, Berglund et al., 2005; Kessler, Chiu et al., 2005).

The *DSM-5* now recognizes agoraphobia as a separate diagnosable disorder, as it can occur without the presence of a panic disorder. Agoraphobia is a low frequency occurrence; an estimated 1.3% of adults may experience the disorder (Kessler, Berglund et al., 2005; Kessler, Chiu et al., 2005). An individual may be diagnosed with agoraphobia if he or she displays extreme fear for at least six months in two of the following situations: (a) leaving the house alone; (b) public transportation; (c) public open spaces; (d) places with no escape or emergency help available in case of a panic attack; and (e) places that ignite anxiety and are avoided or endured with severe anxiety (APA, 2013). The behavior must affect the person's social or occupational functioning. Cultural considerations of this disorder include the relationship of perceived fear to actual fear in the context of the cultural environment.

An individual that displays intense fear toward an object or situation that habitually produces anxiety, and therefore avoids the feared stimuli or endures the anxiety, may be diagnosed with specific phobia (APA, 2013). This disorder is quite common in the general adult population with estimated prevalence rates of 12.5% (Kessler, Berglund et al., 2005; Kessler, Chiu et al., 2005). This consistent fear must last for six months and significantly affect that person's social or occupational functioning. Possible phobic objects or situations may include animals; natural environments such as heights or water; fear of blood, injection, or injury; daily situations such as driving; and other phobic stimuli, such as fear of vomiting. As with other terror stricken anxieties, it is important to consider the client's sociocultural context and assess whether the fear is out of proportion to the actual danger.

Social anxiety disorder is characterized by extreme fear of social situations that may involve scrutiny (APA, 2013). Approximately 12.1% of adults experience a social anxiety that qualifies for diagnosis (Kessler, Berglund et al., 2005; Kessler, Chiu et al., 2005). Typical fearful situations may include conversations with others, being observed while doing a task, or performing a task in front of others. The individual may fear humiliation or rejection due to his or her display of anxious symptoms or performance. For diagnosis, the situation must consistently evoke fear causing the individual to avoid the situation or endure it with extreme anxiety. There are three subtypes of social anxiety disorder, including performance only, generalized, and selective mutism (e.g., the individual does not speak in school, yet speaks at home). As with agoraphobia and specific phobia, the interviewer should assess whether the fear is out of proportion to the actual danger presented in relation to the individual's sociocultural context.

Generalized anxiety disorder is estimated to occur in 5.7% of the adult population at any given point in time (Kessler, Berglund et al., 2005; Kessler, Chiu et al., 2005). An individual may qualify for diagnosis if he exhibits intense worry about two or more aspects of functioning, such as family or work, for three consecutive months (APA, 2013). He must experience physical anxiety symptoms, such as restlessness, fatigue, irritability, and sleep disturbance, and must also exhibit one of the following behaviors: (a) avoid situations that produce anxiety; (b) spend time preparing for these situations; (c) procrastinate due to anxiety; or (d) seek constant reassurance for his excessive worry.

In combination, anxiety disorders are one of the most prevalent mental health disturbances, with studies reporting rates of 10% in children and adolescents and 25% in adults (Esbjorn et al., 2010, Kessler, Berglund et al., 2005; Kessler, Chiu et al., 2005). With youth referred for psychological evaluation, it is estimated that 27–57% are diagnosed with anxiety disorders (Esbjorn et al., 2010). Children with anxiety disorders are also highly likely to maintain the disturbance into adulthood, with studies reporting lifetime prevalence rates of diagnosed children at 29%.

However, many studies report drastic differences in prevalence and comorbidity rates. Possible explanations include the variation in diagnostic instruments used in clinical practice, as well as cultural differences. Individuals in some cultures may not refer individuals with anxious symptoms for psychological evaluation as it is seen as a normal condition in development (Esbjorn et al., 2010). Also, anxious symptoms are likely to appear as physical complaints and may go unrecognized as a manifestation of anxiety, especially in children. With variation in diagnostic procedures across populations, it is important for all clinicians to familiarize themselves with the usefulness, reliability, validity, and limitations of assessment instruments to ensure ethical practice.

HIGHLIGHTS OF FREE-ACCESS INSTRUMENTS USED TO IDENTIFY AND MONITOR OUTCOMES

A variety of instruments are available to measure the presence and severity of anxiety disorders. This section will highlight commonly used free-access instruments for the assessment of anxiety disorders.

HAMILTON ANXIETY SCALE

The Hamilton Anxiety Scale (HAM-A) was designed to assess the severity of anxious symptoms in individuals with neurotic anxiety (Beck & Steer, 1991). It is also referred to as the Hamilton Anxiety Rating Scale (HARS), though this section will refer to it as the HAM-A. While this instrument is intended for use by a skilled clinician, it is also available for free access online at http://www.anxietyhelp.org/information/hama.html?noteListPage=all¬eListSort=¬eListMode=0. Some individuals may wish to use this instrument online prior to seeking mental health assistance.

The HAM-A is a 14-item semi-structured interview instrument. The instrument examines the client's psychic and somatic components of anxiety (Beck & Steer, 1991). The psychic factor assesses anxious mood, tensions, fearfulness, insomnia, intellect/cognitive functioning, depressed mood, and behavior at the interview. The somatic factor assesses muscular, sensory, cardiovascular, respiratory, gastrointestinal, genitourinary, and autonomic symptoms. Clinicians rate interviewee responses on a five point scale ranging from 0 (not present) to 4 (severe). Total scores may range from 0 to 56. Scores of 30 and above denote severe anxiety; 25 to 30, moderate to severe; 18 to 24, mild to moderate; and scores below 17 indicate mild anxiety.

Since its original development in 1959, few studies have examined the psychometric properties of the HAM-A, leaving clinicians and researchers with little information about its validity and usefulness in practice (Maier et al., 1988). Despite this fact, it is commonly used to evaluate the treatment effectiveness of anxiety-reducing drugs. Several versions have been created since 1959; however, the original instrument is most popularly used today.

As it is a clinical interview instrument, the validity and reliability of results depend on the skill level of the administrator as well as influences of the clinician during the interview. Researchers have found interrater reliability among clinicians to be moderate at .73 for psychic ratings, .70 for somatic ratings, and .74 for total scale score (Maier et al., 1988). The Hamilton Anxiety Rating Scale Interview Guide (HARS-IG; Bruss, Gruenberg, Goldstein, & Barber, 1994) is a standardized and structured instrument developed to use in combination with the HAM-A in order to improve reliability. Researchers found interrater reliability coefficients to improve and range from .79 to .81 when used in combination with the HARS-IG. Clinicians should be aware of this limitation and cross validate their conclusions.

The HAM-A has demonstrated adequate score internal consistency with coefficients reported at .79 for the somatic scale and .73 for the psychic scale (Beck & Steer, 1991). Moderate convergent validity was found with the commonly used Beck Anxiety Inventory yielding a coefficient of .56. Strong convergence ($r = .85$) was found with a similar free-access instrument, the GAD-7 (Ruiz et al., 2011). Strong validity and reliability was reported for scores on the Spanish translation of the

HAM-A in use with research and assessment of anxious clients (Lobo et al., 2001).

The HAM-A is a brief and efficient tool to measure anxious symptoms. Researchers have recommended the HAM-A for exploratory purposes as it demonstrates adequate yet not optimal psychometric properties (Beck & Steer, 1991). Researchers also recommend pairing the HAM-A with the HARS-IG for consistent administration results.

Overall Anxiety Severity and Impairment Scale (OASIS)

The OASIS was designed to assess the frequency and severity of an individual's anxiety that has occurred in the past week (Campbell-Sills et al., 2009). This instrument should be used as a screening tool for individuals exhibiting anxious symptoms and experiencing impaired occupational or social functioning. This instrument can be self-administered, for free, online at http://chammp.org/Training/Resources/Assessment-Tools/Anxiety.aspx.

The OASIS is a brief self-report instrument which contains five items. It usually takes less than five minutes to complete. The assessment asks users to respond to the items on a five-point Likert-type scale from 0 to 4 depending on the level of severity perceived for each item. All items are summed to obtain scores ranging from 0 to 20. A score of eight or higher is considered substantial enough to indicate clinical anxiety. Individuals that obtain a cut-off score of eight or above should seek further assessment.

Preliminary psychometric studies have demonstrated reasonable score reliability and validity of the OASIS. High test-retest reliability was found at .82 over a one-month period (Campbell-Sills et al., 2009). OASIS scores showed moderate convergent validity correlations ranging from .4–.6 with similar measures on the BSI-18-A, PDSS, SPIN, GADSS, and the PCL-C. The OASIS also demonstrated moderate correlations ranging from .64–.7 with the BSI-A, TRAIT, SIAS, and NEO-N (Norman et al., 2011). Evidence of divergent validity was shown with NEO-FFI subscales Openness ($r = .07$) and Agreeableness at ($r = -.06$), as well as with the BIS ($r = .09$).

The OASIS is an efficient screening tool for the presence of anxious symptoms. The OASIS is one of the few anxiety assessments that measures life function impairment in addition to physical and cognitive symptoms. A limitation of the instrument is that it only inquires about anxiety related issues that have taken place within the last week, which is inconsistent with current *DSM* criteria. Further research is needed to confirm the validity of the OASIS in diverse populations and settings.

Generalized Anxiety Disorder Screener (GAD-7)

The GAD-7 is a simple instrument designed to assess the presence of generalized anxiety disorder (GAD) symptoms based on criteria listed in the *DSM-IV* (Spitzer, Kroenke, Williams, & Löwe, 2006). It can be accessed, for free, online at http://www.remap.net/GAD_7.html. It is appropriate for use with adults aged 18 years and older.

This self-report instrument contains seven items and should take an individual no longer than five minutes to complete. Items are scored on a four-point scale from 0 (not at all) to 3 (nearly every day). Total scores can range from 0 to 21. Total scores of 0–4 denote minimal or no anxiety while scores of 5–9 indicate mild anxiety, scores of 10–14 moderate anxiety, and scores of 15 and above are considered severe anxiety. A cut-off score of 10 is recommended for further assessment of a possible GAD diagnosis.

Initial studies have demonstrated both the reliability and validity of scores on the GAD-7; however, further research is needed. High internal consistency coefficients have been reported at .89 in the general population and .92 in primary care (Löwe et al., 2008; Spitzer et al., 2006). Scores on the GAD-7 showed moderate convergent validity with like measures of anxiety including the BAI, SCL-90 Anxiety subscale, PHQ-2, and HAM-A (Löwe et al., 2008; Ruiz et al., 2011; Spitzer et al., 2006). The GAD-7 has demonstrated the ability to discriminate between those with generalized anxiety disorder and those without the condition, in primary care (Spitzer et al., 2006). With a cut score of 10, sensitivity and specificity were both reported above .80. Expected gender effects were revealed as women reported elevated levels of anxiety (Löwe et al., 2008).

The GAD-7 should be used as a screening tool, and to assess for severity of GAD. The GAD-7 is extremely brief and can be completed without the assistance of a clinician, rendering it useful for primary care. While this instrument is fairly new, few studies have examined its applicability to diverse populations. Clinicians should be aware of this limitation.

SPENCE CHILDREN'S ANXIETY SCALE

The Spence Children's Anxiety Scale (SCAS) (Spence, 1998) was designed to screen children and adolescents aged eight to 15 years old for anxiety disorders according to the criteria provided in the *DSM-IV*. The instrument may be individually, group, or self-administered online. It should take less than 10 minutes to complete. It can be accessed, for free, online at http://www.scaswebsite.com.

The SCAS contains 44 items, 38 of which are related to the six categories of anxiety disorders. The remaining six items are positive fillers to prevent negative response bias. Clients respond to items on a four-point Likert-type scale ranging from 0 to 3: never (0), sometimes (1), often (2), and always (3). All items, except for numbers 11, 17, 26, 31, 38, and 43, which are the positive filler items, are summed and can be converted to T scores (http://www.scaswebsite.com/). The maximum score possible is 114. T scores of 60 or higher may indicate the presence of an anxiety disorder. Interpretations of scores are separated for gender and age groups: 8–11 years and 12–15 years. T score conversion charts are provided on the website.

To supplement the SCAS, a parent version (SCAS-P) of the instrument was developed, asking parents about observable anxious behaviors in their child. The SCAS-P maintains a similar structure, with 38 items without the positive filler items. A parent report for preschool children was also developed to assist in identifying children at risk of developing anxiety disorders (Spence, Rapee, McDonald, & Ingram, 2001). Researchers proposed the need for direct behavioral measures in addition to parent observation.

The SCAS has demonstrated reasonable psychometric properties. Internal consistency was reportedly .93. Test-retest reliability was moderate at .63 for 12 weeks and .60 for six months (Spence, 1998; Spence, Barrett, & Turner, 2003). The SCAS scores showed high convergent validity ranging from .70–.75 with related criterion measures on the Revised Children's Manifest Anxiety Scale. A moderate correlation ($r = .60$) was reported with the Child Depression Inventory. Researchers found strong support for the six-correlated-factor model, which included separation anxiety, social phobia, obsessive-compulsive disorder, panic/agoraphobia, physical injury fears, and generalized anxiety (Spence, 1997). Significant gender effects were found (Spence, 1998). Girls reported significantly higher scores than males across ages. Younger children reported higher scores than older children across gender. SCAS-P scores also demonstrated adequate internal reliability (.89) and strong evidence for convergent and divergent validity (Nauta et al., 2004).

The SCAS has shown adequate reliability and validity as a screening tool for children in research and clinical use. The SCAS is also appropriate for use as a measurement for severity of anxious symptoms and to monitor treatment outcomes. A revised edition will be needed to align with the *DSM-5*, as obsessive compulsive behavior is no longer categorized as an anxiety disorder.

Social Phobia Inventory (SPIN)

The SPIN can be accessed online at http://psychology-tools.com/spin. The SPIN was developed as a self-assessment tool to measure severity of social phobia. The instrument evaluates the experience of fear, avoidance, and physiological discomfort in relation to authority, parties, criticism, strangers, being watched, or embarrassment. The SPIN should take less than 10 minutes to complete.

The SPIN contains 17 items which assess fear of authority, parties, criticism, strangers, being watched, or embarrassment; avoidance of talking to others or speaking around others, parties, attention, speeches, criticism, and speaking to authority; and physiological discomfort such as blushing, sweating, or shaking in front of others (Connor et al., 2000). Items are scored on a five-point Likert-type scale ranging from 0 to 4: not at all (0), a little bit (1), somewhat (2), very much (3), and extremely (4). All items are summed for a total score. Total scores can range from 0 to 68. A cut-off total score of 19 or higher indicates a clinically significant level of social phobia.

Psychometric properties of the SPIN have shown adequate support for its use. Strong internal consistency coefficients have been reported from .82–.94 (Connor et al., 2000). Antony, Coons, McCabe, Ashbaugh, & Swinson (2006) found internal consistencies for each subscale at .85 for fear, .82 for avoidance, and .79 for physiological in those diagnosed with social phobia. Test-retest reliability has been moderate to strong with coefficients ranging from .78–.89 (Antony et al., 2006; Connor et al., 2000). The SPIN displayed convergent validity with the BSPS at .57–.80, CSAS at .55, and FQ social phobia subscale at .77 (Connor et al., 2000). Significant concordance was also found with the Social Phobia Scale at .71 and the Social Interaction Anxiety Scale at .60 (Antony et al., 2006). Divergent validity was found with the general health scale on the SF-36. With a cut-off score of 19, the SPIN demonstrated 79% diagnostic accuracy in identifying those with or without social phobia (Connor et al., 2000). The SPIN successfully discriminated between those with social phobia and other anxiety disorders (Antony et al., 2006). The SPIN also demonstrated strong ability to discriminate between different treatments' effectiveness (Connor et al., 2000; Antony et al., 2006).

The SPIN should be used for individual assessment for severity of social phobia symptomology and to monitor the efficacy of treatments. The SPIN has yet to be validated using diverse populations. Clinicians should be aware of this limitation and use caution when using the SPIN with children or ethnic populations.

CHAPTER 3

Assessment of Mood Disorders

PRIMARY MOOD DISORDERS COMMONLY ENCOUNTERED IN CLINICAL PRACTICE

Mood disorders are commonly experienced in children, adolescents, and adults, and cause significant impairments in life functioning. The most recent edition of the *Diagnostic and Statistical Manual of Mental Disorders* (*DSM-5*; APA, 2013) has separated mood disorders into two categories: depressive disorders, and bipolar and related disorders. The most commonly encountered mood disorders include major depressive disorder (single and recurrent episodes), chronic depressive disorder (previously dysthymia), bipolar disorders I and II, and cyclothymic disorder. Other disorders include disruptive mood dysregulation, premenstrual dysphoric, mixed anxiety/depression, substance-induced depressive, and substance-induced bipolar.

Major depressive disorder may include a single episode or recurrent episodes. A major depressive episode occurs during a two-week period in which the individual experiences symptoms related to either depressed mood or loss of interest or pleasure. The individual must exhibit five or more of the following symptoms: (a) depressed mood throughout the day; (b) decreased pleasure or interest in daily activities; (c) significant weight loss or gain; (d) restlessness or oversleeping; (e) visible psychomotor distress; (f) noticeable decrease in vigor; (g) sense of worthlessness or incongruous guilt; (h) trouble focusing; or (i) fixation with death, suicidal thoughts with or without a plan, or suicidal attempt (APA, 2013).

A diagnosis of major depressive disorder (single episode) is characterized by: (a) the occurrence of one major depressive episode; (b) the episode is not best accounted for by another disorder; and (c) absence of a history of a manic or hypomanic episode. The clinician should specify the current status of the disorder as mild, moderate, or severe, and whether the presence of mood congruent or incongruent psychotic symptoms exists. For a diagnosis of major depressive disorder (recurrent episodes), the criteria are the same, except that the presence of two or more major depressive episodes must exist.

Dysthymic disorder is characterized by depressed mood for most of the day on a majority of days for two years in adults and one year in children and adolescents (APA, 2013). An individual must exhibit two or more of the following symptoms: (a) lack of eating or overeating; (b) restlessness or oversleeping; (c) exhaustion; (d) low sense of confidence; (e) highly distractible; or (f) feelings of despair. For diagnosis, the symptoms must not be absent for more than two months, must not occur with a psychotic disorder, must not be a side effect of a substance, and must cause significant life impairment. Early onset of chronic depressive disorder is considered prior to 21 years and late onset older than 21 years.

Bipolar I disorder consists of four subtypes which pertain to the current or most recent episode, including hypomanic, manic, depressed, or unspecified (APA, 2013). A hypomanic episode is characterized by an elevated irritable mood or increased energy for four days in a row. Criteria for a hypomanic episode includes: (a) occurrence of three or more of the following in the state of increased activity and four or more for irritable mood: exaggerated sense of grandeur, restlessness, unusual garrulousness, racing thoughts, difficulty concentrating, rise in intentional actions or psychomotor disturbance, or indulgence in gratifying activities that have potential adverse effects; (b) the change is incompatible with their personality; (c) the change is noticeable to others; (d) the behavior does not involve psychotic symptoms and is not severe enough to cause hospitalization; and (e) the behavior is not due to another substance (APA, 2013). Bipolar II disorder (current or most recent episode hypomanic) is diagnosable if the most recent or current episode is hypomanic, a manic episode has occurred previously, it causes significant impairment in life functioning, and is not best accounted for by a personality disorder. The clinician should also specify features of the disorder which may include psychotic, mixed, catatonic, rapid cycling, anxiety, suicide risk severity, or seasonal pattern.

A manic episode consists of the same criteria as a hypomanic episode, with the exception of the duration, which must last one week (APA, 2013). Bipolar I disorder (current or most recent episode manic) is characterized by the presence of a most recent or current manic episode, history of a previous manic episode, and the behaviors must not be best accounted for by another personality disorder. Features of the disorder are the same as hypomanic with the addition of postpartum onset.

Bipolar I disorder (current or most recent episode depressed) is characterized by the presence of a current or most recent major depressive episode, history of a previous manic episode, and the symptoms are not best accounted for by another disorder (APA, 2013). For diagnosis, the individual must exhibit three symptoms of a major depressive episode, and one symptom must be depressed mood or anhedonia. The clinician should specify features of the disorder, which are the same as hypomanic with the addition of melancholic and atypical features. The fourth subtype, unspecified, is diagnosable if the individual meets all the criteria except for the duration for a manic, hypomanic, or depressive episode; a previous history of a manic episode has occurred; the disturbance causes significant life impairment; and symptoms are not better accounted for by another disorder.

Bipolar II disorder has two subtypes: hypomanic and depressed. Current or most recent episode hypomanic is characterized by a history (a) of one or more major depressive episodes; (b) of one hypomanic episode; (c) absent a manic episode; (d) of symptoms not better accounted for by another personality disorder; and which (e) causes significant life functioning impairment (APA, 2013). The clinician should also specify features of the disorder, which may include psychotic, mixed, rapid cycling, anxiety, suicide risk severity, seasonal pattern, or postpartum onset. Current or most recent episode depressed comprises the same criteria with depressed behavior as the prominent presentation. Features of the disorder include psychotic, mixed, catatonic, rapid cycling, anxiety, suicide risk severity, seasonal pattern, melancholic, atypical features, or postpartum onset.

Cyclothymic disorder is characterized by: (a) two years of prolonged hypomanic and depressive periods in adults and one year in children and adolescents (the criteria for hypomanic episode is met, but major depressive episode criteria is not met); (b) during the initial onset, symptoms have not been absent for more than two months at a time; (c) absence of major depressive or manic episodes during the initial onset; (d) symptoms are not better accounted for by another disorder; (e) symptoms are not a result of substances; and (e) the behaviors must significantly impair life functioning (APA, 2013). Features of the disorder include mixed, rapid, anxiety, suicide risk severity, seasonal pattern, and postpartum onset.

Disruptive mood dysregulation disorder is a newly proposed disorder in the most recent edition of the *DSM*. It is characterized by excessive verbal or behavioral temper outbursts that are inappropriate for an individual's developmental age and which are followed by a consistent negative mood (APA, 2013). The symptoms must occur three times per week in two or more settings for more than 12 months, and must not be absent for more than three consecutive months. Children are eligible at six years old for diagnosis, but onset must occur prior to ten years of age. Behavioral display of this disorder must not occur during a psychotic episode or as a characteristic of a mood disorder; however, it may be comorbid with attention-deficit/hyperactivity disorder, oppositional defiant disorder, or conduct disorder.

Premenstrual dysmorphic disorder is also a new proposal for the latest edition. For diagnosis, the characteristic symptoms must occur mainly during the week before menses and must subside for the most part thereafter (APA, 2013). The following four symptoms must be present: (a) intense change in affect (sudden sadness or mood swings); (b) increased anger or conflicts; (c) significant display of depressed mood and feelings of hopelessness; and (d) increased anxiety or tension. In addition to the previous symptoms, one or more of the following symptoms must also occur: loss of interest in usual activities; fatigue; change in eating habits; insomnia or hypersomnia; feeling out of control; or physical symptoms, such as bloating or muscle pain.

Mixed anxiety/depression is a new disorder proposed to focus treatment and aid effectiveness, as anxiety often occurs with depression but may not meet criteria for diagnosis (APA, 2013). The criteria of this disorder involve three to four major depressive symptoms combined with anxious distress for two weeks. Anxious distress is defined as irrational or excessive worry and preoccupation with worries, difficulty relaxing, muscle tension, and fear of an impending negative event.

Substance-induced depressive and bipolar disorders comprise similar criteria. The depressive or bipolar behaviors must occur during or after one month of severe intoxication or withdrawal. The disorders must cause significant life impairment and must not have occurred prior to the substance use.

A depressive and bipolar condition not elsewhere classified consists of presentations of the disorders which may not meet the criteria according to duration or number of symptoms required. Unspecified depressive or bipolar disorders are also options for those who do not meet specific criteria, yet still warrant clinical attention. Depressive or bipolar disorders may also present with a known general medical condition.

Mood disorders are the most commonly experienced mental health disturbance in the general population. In the United States, combined prevalence for major depression, dysthymic disorder, and bipolar disorder has been estimated at 9.5% for adults (Kessler, Chiu, Demler, & Walters, 2005). In adolescents aged 13–18 years, lifetime prevalence has been estimated at 14% (Merikangas et al., 2010). A lack of adequate data has been available regarding the occurrence of mood disorders in children younger than 13 years. In both adolescents and adults, estimated prevalence is higher in females than males.

Major depression is one of the most debilitating health conditions that affect all ages and ethnicities (González, Tarraf, Whitfield & Vega, 2010). Prevalence for 12-month diagnosis in U.S. adults has been estimated at 6.7%, with higher rates reported in women (Kessler, Chiu et al., 2005). Major depression has high comorbidity rates with anxiety disorders and high recurrence rates for 12-month diagnosis (Kessler et al., 2003). Lifetime prevalence rates have been estimated to range from 16.2%-18.6% in the general adult population, with varying rates among age groups, socioeconomic statuses, and ethnicities (Gonzalez et al., 2010; Kessler et al., 2003; Kessler, Berglund et al., 2005). In adolescents aged 13–18 years, lifetime prevalence rates for major depression and dysthmic disorder were combined and estimated at 11.2% with higher rates reported for females (Merikangas et al., 2010).

In comparison to major depression, occurrence of dysthmia and bipolar disorder in U.S. adults is infrequent. Prevalence for dysthmia has been reported at 1.5% for 12-month diagnosis and 2.5% for lifetime diagnosis (Kessler, Berglund et al., 2005; Kessler, Chiu et al., 2005). Prevalence for 12-month diagnosis of bipolar disorder has been estimated at 2.6% and lifetime diagnoses are estimated at 3.9% (Kessler, Berglund et al., 2005; Kessler, Chiu et al., 2005). Incidence of bipolar disorder in children and adolescents was estimated between zero and 3%; however, researchers and clinicians have expressed concerns about appropriate guidelines for diagnosis in those aged 18 years and younger.

Given the pervasiveness of mood disorders in the general population, it is essential for clinicians to identify those in need of assistance. Of those with a reported mood disorder, 56.4% sought services for treatment (Wang et al., 2005). However, only 38.3% reported adequate treatment for their disorder. Clinicians must become aware of psychometrically sound screening and diagnostic tools to best assess the clients' needs and provide sufficient treatment for relief of their disorder.

Highlights of Free-access Instruments Used to Identify and Monitor Outcomes

There are several assessment tools available to assess the presence and severity of specific mood disorders. This section will highlight some of the most commonly used free-access instruments for self or clinician use.

Hamilton Rating Scale for Depression

The Hamilton Rating Scale for Depression is a self-report instrument designed to evaluate the severity of symptoms in those diagnosed with a depressive disorder (Hamilton, 1960). It is also referred to as the Hamilton Depression Scale, and is commonly abbreviated to HAM-D and the HRSD. The HAM-D has been considered the gold standard in evaluating the effectiveness of antidepressants in clinical trials and has been widely used since its development in 1960 (Bagby, Ryder, Schuller, & Marshall, 2004). While multiple versions of the scale exist, this review will focus on the original 17-item structure, as it is used most frequently. The HAM-D can be accessed, for free, online at https://www.outcometracker.org/library/HAM-D.pdf.

The HAM-D self-report instrument may take 15 to 20 minutes to complete and should be administered individually. The HAM-D performs best when paired with a structured interview administered by trained clinicians (Carmody et al., 2006). The self-report instrument contains 17 items designed to assess depressive symptomology. Hamilton (1960) developed the instrument to assess 10 variables of depression. The following eight variables ask respondents to rate their experience on a five-point Likert-type scale from 0–4 with higher ratings indicating severe symptoms: dejected mood; feelings of inappropriate guilt; thoughts of suicide; disinterest or disengagement in daily activities; psychomotor delay; psychological anxiety; physical anxiety; and preoccupation with health. The following eight variables ask respondents to rate their experience using a three-point Likert-type scale from 0–2 with higher ratings indicating severe symptoms: trouble falling asleep; insomnia during the night; early morning insomnia; visible physical tension; gastro-intestinal complaints; general somatic indicators; genital issues; and awareness of condition. A two-part variable asks respondents to rate the severity of their weight loss history and current status on a three-point scale from 0–2.

Items are summed for a total score. Raw scores may range from 0 to 52. Hamilton suggested that two raters should score patient responses for maximum reliability. Interpretation of scores for the original 17-item HAM-D with score range of 0 to 52 are categorized as the following: 0–7, not depressed; 8–12, minor depression; 13–17, less than major depression; 18–29, major depression; and 30–31 or greater, severe depression (Kriston & von Wolff, 2011). Interpretations for other versions of the instrument vary in the literature. Cut-off scores for signs of major depressive disorder remission have been recommended at less than or equal to seven. However, recent research suggests that a true indication of return to normal and occupational functioning should be less than or equal to five (Romera, Pérez, Menchón, Polavieja, & Gilaberte, 2011).

Studies examining the psychometric properties of the HAM-D have reported mixed results. While the HAM-D has shown adequate score reliability and validity, argument exists over the design of the instrument. Researchers argued that the items measure multiple constructs, leading to an unclear interpretation of the total score (Bagby et al., 2004;

Carmody et al., 2006). This multidimensionality has prevented agreement on a unifying factor structure, as many studies report a varying number of factors. The instrument also lacks coincidence with *DSM-IV* criteria. Researchers suggested the need to recreate the instrument to fix inherent errors in the original item structure and update the content to match current depression criteria.

Scores on the HAM-D have shown high reliability. Trajković et al. (2011) conducted a meta-analysis including 49 years of studies on the HAM-D and found strong evidence of reliability with mean correlation coefficients of .79 for internal consistency, .93 for interrater reliability, and .87 for test-retest reliability. Bagby et al. (2004) conducted a review of studies from 1980 to 2003 that reported total item correlation coefficients ranging from .46 to .97 for internal reliability, .82–.98 for interrater reliability, and .81–.98 for test-retest reliability. However, individual item correlations were weak, which suggested errors with several items. In an effort to improve reliability, the Structured Interview Guide for the Hamilton Depression Rating Scale (SIGH-D) was developed to establish standardization in administration of the instrument (Williams, 1988).

HAM-D scores showed strong convergent validity with several measures of depression. Convergence with the Beck Depression Inventory (BDI) in clinical adult populations was shown with coefficients of .70 at one month and .85 at eight months in agreement with patient symptom severity (Brown, Schulberg, & Madonia, 1995). Bagby et al. (2004) found correlations with the BDI ranging from .48 to .89. Correlations with the Montgomery Äsberg Rating Scale of Depression (MADRS) were found at .88 and .92 with two different populations (Carmody et al., 2006). A lack of convergent validity was found with the Structured Clinical Interview for *DSM-IV* (SCID-I). Bagby et al. concluded that the instrument needed updated item content to correspond with current diagnostic criteria. Pancheri, Picardi, Pasquini, Gaetano, & Biondi (2002) also found the instrument to lack the dimension of hyperactivation in depression.

The HAM-D demonstrated strong discriminant validity. In the geriatric population, the instrument obtained high accuracy rates in identifying individuals with depression (Mottram, Wilson, & Copeland, 2000). Using a cut-off score of 16, researchers reported sensitivity at .88 and specificity at .99, as well as positive predictive value at .99 and negative predictive value at .97. The instrument has shown its ability to successfully discriminate between healthy, depressed, and bipolar patients; with bipolar patients scoring highest (Rehm & O'Hara, 1985). The HAM-D scores also showed discriminant validity among mild, moderate, and severely depressed patients (Zheng et al., 1988).

Argument exists over a universal factor structure of the HAM-D. The scale is multidimensional and studies have disagreed over the optimal factor structure, with number of factors ranging from two to eight (Bagby et al., 2004). One study reported a reliable four-factor structure - including somatic anxiety, hypochondriasis, general somatic symptoms, and insomnia - which accounted for 43.8% of the total variance (Pancheri et al., 2002). Carmody et al. (2006) reported a two-factor model, with six to seven items failing to fit the model. A six-factor structure accounted for 55.4% of the total variance on the following factors: anxiety, weight loss, depression, health concerns, sleep/libido, and anhedonia/energy (Brown et al., 1995). In light of the disagreement on one-factor structure, researchers cautioned users to recognize the multidimensionality of the scale and interpret results accordingly (Pancheri et al., 2002).

The HAM-D should be used for evaluation of depression severity for those previously diagnosed with a depressive disorder. Information gleaned from the HAM-D can be useful in treatment planning and evaluating treatment effectiveness. The HAM-D is advantageous for clinicians and research as it produces a multidimensional assessment of depression. However, the HAM-D may not be most cost effective, as it is time consuming and should be administered by trained clinicians and paired with a structured interview. Researchers have advocated for the recreation of the HAM-D items to eliminate the assessment of multiple constructs and to coincide with current diagnostic criteria. Users should be aware of the limitations of this instrument and use caution in interpretation and generalization.

Center for Epidemiologic Studies—Depression

The Center for Epidemiologic Studies–Depression (CES-D) is a self-report inventory used to screen for depressive symptoms that have occurred during the past week in non-psychiatric populations (Van Dam & Earleywine, 2011). The instrument was originally developed to assess symptom severity in adults and has since been modified for use with adolescents (Santor, Zuroff, Ramsay, Cervantes, & Palacios, 1995). This instrument can be accessed online at http://www.chcr.brown.edu/pcoc/cesdscale.pdf

The CES-D contains 20 items which correspond with the *DSM-IV* criteria for depressive disorders. The instrument may be self or clinician-administered and should take no longer than five minutes to complete (Radloff, 1977). The items pertain to general depression characteristics including depressed mood, feelings of guilt or worthlessness, feelings of helplessness or hopelessness, and somatic complaints (Carlson et al., 2011). Clients are asked to respond to items on a four-point scale based on the frequency with which they have experienced the symptoms. Ratings range from 0 to 3: "rarely, less than one day" (0); "some or little of the time, one to two days (1); "occasionally or a moderate amount of time, three to four days" (2); and "most all of the time, five to seven days" (3). Four items are reverse scored and aim to measure the absence of a positive outlook.

Item responses are summed for a total score. Scores may range from 0 to 60 (Radloff, 1977). Radloff originally proposed that scores of 16 or above denoted severe cases of depression. Santor et al. (1995) confirmed the accuracy of this cut-off point in adults, yet cautioned that it may result in over identification of adolescents and should be higher.

The CES-D has shown reasonable score validity and reliability. Internal consistency reports for non-reverse scored items ranged from .73–.88 (Carlson et al., 2011; Stommel et al., 1993). Internal consistency correlations for reverse scored items were .67 (Carlson et al., 2011). Mean item correlations for reverse and non-reverse scored items were moderate with correlations of .45 and .59 respectively. Van Dam and Earleywine (2011) found moderate correlations with the STICSA, .65–.74 and the PANAS, .58. However, low convergence was found with the SPQ-B, .43–.44 (Santor et al., 1995).

Since its original development, a four-factor model has been proposed and confirmed to best fit the CES-D data (Hertzog, Van Alstine, Usala, Hultsch, & Dixon, 1990; Knight, Williams, McGee, & Olaman, 1997). The four-factor structure includes depressive mood, well-being, somatic symptoms, and interpersonal (Stommel et al., 1993). However, debate exists over the plausibility of a single or two-factor model compared to a four-factor structure. Van Dam and Earlywine (2011) proposed that a single-factor model best fits the data with two main symptom clusters related to negative mood and functional impairment. Edwards, Cheavens, Heiy, and Cukrowicz (2010) suggested that, while a four-factor model fits the data, a two-factor model fits the data as well. Edwards et al. recommended that a one-factor model does not fit the data best, but should be used for interpretation as it is the most reasonable structure. Recommendations for future research suggest the separation of the four reverse scored items for scoring purposes and for a single-factor model fit.

Despite reports on adequate psychometric properties for total scores, few individual items lack adequate reliability and validity due to item response bias. Researchers have reported that two items produced racial response bias (Cole, Kawachi, Maller, & Berkman, 2000; Yang & Jones, 2007). Black respondents consistently scored higher on the items "people are unfriendly" and "people dislike me" than their white counterparts. Researchers reported gender response bias for the items which contained "crying" and "talked less" (Cole et al. 2000; Stommel et al., 1993; Yang & Jones, 2007). Women consistently produced higher scores for "crying" while men consistently produced higher scores for "talked less," as they are gender specific features of depression. Several studies have also found a cultural response bias in ethnic populations, which were a majority Asian, as they overinflated responses on positively worded items, likely due to cultural expectations (Demirchyan, Petrosyan, & Thompson, 2011; Lee, J. J., et al., 2011; Li & Hicks, 2010).

Strommel et al. (1993) proposed the removal of the interpersonal items as they are not measures of depression. Strommel et al. also suggested removing the gender bias response items - "crying", "talked less", and "thought life a failure" items - and recommended the need for a 15-item instrument. The 15-item structure demonstrated high internal reliability (.88) and strong concurrent validity of .98 with the 20-item structure.

The CES-D is widely used in assessment of depression in the general population. While adequate psychometric properties have been demonstrated, several items have shown item response bias for race, gender, and culture. Lack of individual item reliability has likely resulted in the disagreement on factor structure. Researchers have proposed removal of these items to enhance validity and reliability across populations. Clinicians should be aware of these limitations and only use the instrument for screening in populations in which the CES-D has been validated.

THE SCHEDULE FOR AFFECTIVE DISORDERS AND SCHIZOPHRENIA FOR SCHOOL-AGE CHILDREN

The Schedule for Affective Disorders and Schizophrenia for School-Age Children (K-SADS) is a semi-structured clinical interview designed to screen children aged six to 18 years for the presence of affective disorders and schizophrenia (Birmaher et al., 2009). Several versions of the diagnostic interview exist including Present State (K-SADS-P), Epidemiologic (K-SADS-E), and Present and Lifetime (K-SADS-PL) (Ambrosini, 2000). The K-SADS-P rates the frequency and severity of symptomology from the previous year as well as the current episode. The K-SADS-E indicates the presence or absence of symptoms in past severe episodes and rates the severity of symptoms during the current episode. The K-SADS-PL extends upon the K-SADS-P as it inquires about lifetime psychopathology and includes screening items for 32 *DSM-IV* Axis I diagnoses (Kaufman et al., 1997). The K-SADS-PL is available, for free, online at http://www.wpic.pitt.edu/research/AssessmentTools/ChildAdolescent/ksads-pl.pdf.

The K-SADS-PL must be administered by a trained clinician. It is given to both the parent and child to assess the presence or absence of *DSM-IV* symptomology (Kaufman et al., 1997). In the general population, the parent and child interviews should take 35 to 45 minutes. However, in the psychiatric population, interviews may take 75 minutes each. When administered to children, the parent is interviewed first; however, with adolescents, the parent is interviewed second. The K-SADS-PL contains several components for a full assessment beginning with an Introductory Interview, followed by the Screen Interview, and ending with the Diagnostic Supplement.

The Introductory Interview should take 10 to 15 minutes to complete and inquires about the client's psychological, medical, and social history, as well as current functioning (Kaufman et al., 1997). The Screen Interview contains items which assess the presence of 82 symptoms in 20 diagnostic areas. Children and parents respond to interview questions and the clinician rates responses on a four-point scale according to (0) insignificant information available; (1) symptomology not present; (2)

sub-threshold presentation of symptoms; and (3) threshold presentation of symptom criteria. Several questions are scored on a three-point scale with the following designations: (0) not enough information; (1) not present; and (2) present.

Responses from the child and parent are recorded on a single sheet to compare answers. If the client does not present significant symptomology, then the client meets "skip-out" criteria and the clinician skips the remaining questions for the diagnostic category. If the screen is positive, follow-up questions are administered using the Diagnostic Supplement portion to assess five diagnostic categories: (1) affective disorders; (2) psychotic disorders; (3) anxiety disorders; (4) behavior disorders; and (5) substance abuse, eating, and tic disorders. As it is a semi-structured interview, questions asked may vary according to clients' responses. If any inconsistencies between the child and parent reports exist, the clinician may interview them both together to clarify (Ambrosini, 2000). The clinician summarizes the responses with more weight given to observable behaviors rated by the parents and subjective experiences of the child. The clinician summary is interpreted for diagnosis and treatment planning.

The K-SADS-PL has demonstrated strong psychometric properties. Researchers have confirmed score reliability and validity in the school-age population it was designed for, and recent evidence suggests its use with preschool-aged children (Birmaher et al., 2009; Kaufman et al., 1997). Reliability scores for the "skip-out," screening, and diagnostic portions are reported separately. Interrater agreement for the "skip-out" portion is reported at 99.7% (Kaufman et al., 1997). "Skip-out" test-retest reliabilities were moderate to strong, with kappas ranging from .52 to .80. Interrater agreement for present and lifetime diagnoses was 98%. Test-retest reliability for diagnosis was moderate to strong, with coefficients ranging from .60 to 1.00 for present and lifetime diagnosis. The lowest score was reported at .55 for AD/HD. In support of concurrent validity, depressive scores correlated highly with the CBCL–Internalizing Scale; anxiety scores with the SCARED for Children and Parents and CBCL–Externalizing Scale; and AD/HD scores correlated highly with the Conner's Parent Rating Scale.

The K-SADS is a comprehensive and efficient tool to screen and diagnose a broad range of *DSM-IV* Axis I Disorders in children and adolescents. The screen interview and use of "skip-out" criteria of the K-SADS-PL shorten administration time, which renders it useful for research and clinical populations While the K-SADS-PL assesses additional disorders compared to the K-SADS-P and K-SADS-E, the dichotomous nature lacks assessment of symptom severity. Although psychometric evidence supports high interrater agreement for screening and diagnosis, the inherent drawback of the K-SADS-PL is reliance on clinician skill in differential diagnosis. However, the K-SADS-PL is the only version available for free use online.

The Edinburgh Depression Scale

The Edinburgh Depression Scale (EDS), also referred to as the Edinburgh Postnatal Depression Scale (EPDS), is a self-report instrument designed to screen for depression during the postpartum period. The EDS should be used to assess depressive symptomology and identify those at risk of developing postpartum depression (Dennis, 2004). It should not be used as a diagnostic tool. The instrument is available for use online at http://www.valueoptions.com/members/files/Post_Partum_Depression_Screen_(Edinburgh_Post_Natal_Depression_Scale).pdf and at http://fcmc.weebly.com/uploads/3/4/8/9/3489838/edinburghscale.pdf.

The EDS should take less than five minutes to complete, as it is comprised of 10 items. Respondents rate their subjective experience of the severity and frequency of depressive symptoms within the past week. Items 1, 2, and 4 require respondents to rate their experience on a four-point scale of 0–3 with higher numbers denoting increased severity. Items 3 and 5–10 are reverse scored from 3 to 0. Scores are summed for a total score that can range from 0 to 30. Scores of 10 or above denote possible depression. Scores of 12 and above require diagnostic assessment for presence of a clinical disorder.

The EDS has shown adequate concurrent validity with similar measures of depression and anxiety. Coefficients were reported at .75 with the STAI and .59 with the NADJ (Green, 1998). Researchers have argued that the EDS should be a screening measure of dsyphoria, rather than clinical depression, as it also emits a dimension of anxiety.

The EDS has demonstrated satisfactory discriminant validity in several countries and in several different languages with postpartum populations (Benvenuti, Ferrara, Niccolai, Valoriana, & Cox, 1999; Dennis, 2004; Ji et al., 2011; Pitanupong, Liabsuetrakul, & Vittayanont, 2007; Reighard & Evans, 1995; Su et al., 2007; Werrett & Clifford, 2006). In its original development, a cut-off score of 12 was recommended. Recent studies found that a cut-off score of 12/13 produced high sensitivity (93.9%) yet moderate specificity (76.7%), whereas a cut-off score of 9/10 produced high sensitivity (82.9%) and high specificity (86.2%) (Dennis, 2004). The EDS also demonstrated success in predicting postpartum depression at four and eight weeks when the instrument was completed at one week postpartum (Chabrol & Teissedre, 2004; Dennis, 2004).

The EDS scores also showed adequate discriminant validity across perinatal periods including preconception through late postpartum (Ji et al., 2011). Ranges of sensitivity measures were reported at 76% to 87.2% and specificity ranged from 69.9% to 98.5%. Lowest accuracy rates were reported during the early postpartum period. Optimal cut-off scores were found to range considerably during different perinatal periods, with higher scores for earlier stages. As the instrument was designed for the postpartum period, optimal cut-off scores were found at scores of 11 for early postpartum and 12 for late postpartum, with a mean sensitivity rate of 81.3% and specificity rate of 79.1%. Researchers suggest establishing separate cut-off points for different periods of the pregnancy and postpartum period (Ji et al., 2011; Su et al., 2007).

Originally developed to assess postpartum depression in women, studies have shown that new fathers may also experience symptoms of postpartum depression. A recent study suggests the plausibility of the EDS in screening postpartum depression in men, as clinically depressed fathers scored higher than non-depressed fathers (Edmonson, Psychogiou, Vlachos, Netsi, & Ramchandani, 2010). Researchers found that a cut-off score of 10 was best suited for males with 89.5% sensitivity and 78.2% specificity.

The EDS is an efficient screening tool for symptoms of postpartum depression. It demonstrated score validity across perinatal periods for detection and prediction of depression in mothers. The EDS also showed promise for detecting postpartum depression in fathers. The brevity of the instrument is ideal for using in busy health care settings to obtain information for further assessment as needed.

Zung Self-Rating Depression Scale

The Zung Self-Rating Depression Scale (SDS) is a self-report instrument designed to assess the severity of a major depressive episode in the clinical population (Campo-Arias, Díaz-Martínez, Rueda-Jaimes, del Pilar Cadena & Hernández, 2006). It can be accessed, for free, online at http://www.psychology.com/assessments/assessment_start.php?p=1. The instrument is appropriate for use with adults aged 18 years and older.

The SDS contains 20 Likert-type scale items (Campo-Arias et al., 2006). Respondents rate their subjective experience of the item according to a four-point scale: 1 = none or a little of the time, 2 = some of the time, 3 = good part of the time, and 4 = most or all of the time. Responses are assigned scores one to four for the ten positively scored items and four to one for the ten negatively scored items. Item scores are summed and total scores can range from 20 to 80. Scores of 50 to 59 denote symptom severity which may indicate mild to moderate depression, 60–69 may indicate moderate to severe depression, and 70 or above may indicate severe depression (Gabrys & Peters, 1985).

Scores on the SDS were reported as both valid and reliable. The SDS demonstrated high interrater reliability at .89 and high internal reliability coefficients at .82–.93 (de Jonghe & Baneke, 1989; Gabrys & Peters, 1985). Split-half reliability coefficients were reported at .79–.94. The SDS showed convergent validity with the depression scale of the MMPI with a correlation coefficient of .77 in a depressed population (Thurber, Snow, & Honts, 2002). Researchers have supported the original three-factor structure proposed, which includes affective, cognitive, and somatic variables (Kitamura, Hirano, Chen, & Hirata, 2004; Zung, Richards, & Short,1965).

SDS scores demonstrated the ability to discriminate between depressed and non-depressed individuals (de Jonghe & Baneke, 1989; Gabrys & Peters, 1985). False negatives of depressed individuals with scores of 50 or less were reported at 6–8%. In a Columbian community sample, high discriminant validity was found using a cut-off score of 40 (Campo-Arias et al., 2006). Sensitivity was 88.6%, specificity 74.8%, positive predictive power 41.1%, and negative predictive power 97.1%. In a sample of individuals diagnosed with depression and alcohol abuse, using a cut-off score of 50 resulted in 57% sensitivity, 83% specificity, 75%

positive predictive power, and 68% negative predictive power (Thurber et al. 2002).

The SDS is a valid tool to quantify depressive symptom severity in clinical and community populations. The SDS should not be used for diagnosis but should be used to refer clients for further evaluation based on the presentation of symptom severity. Clinicians should establish an appropriate cut-off score that results in high sensitivity and specificity for the client population.

Mood Disorder Questionnaire

The Mood Disorder Questionnaire (MDQ) was developed to screen for bipolar spectrum disorders, which include bipolar I and II, cyclothymia, and bipolar not otherwise specified (Hirschfeld et al., 2000). The MDQ is a patient report instrument, which assesses the lifetime presence or absence of manic and hypomanic symptoms and their impairment on functioning. The instrument can be accessed, for free, online at http://www.dbsalliance.org/pdfs/MDQ.pdf.

The MDQ should take no longer than five minutes to complete. Clients are simply asked to respond "yes" or "no" to 13 symptom items related to manic or hypomanic behavior according to *DSM-IV* criteria (Hirschfeld et al., 2000). The following item asks clients to respond "yes" or "no" to whether any of the above symptoms have occurred at the same time. Next, clients are asked to rate the impact of any of the above symptoms on functioning on a four-point scale: no problem (0), minor problem (1), moderate problem (2), and serious problem (3). Last, the instrument asks clients to indicate whether family or personal history of bipolar disorder exists. Items with a response of "yes" are summed for a total score.

Scores on the MDQ have demonstrated adequate psychometric properties. Hirschfeld et al. found that the optimal cut-off was seven or higher in a psychiatric outpatient population. Sensitivity was reported at .73 and specificity at .90. This indicates that the MDQ correctly identified seven out of 10 individuals who had a bipolar spectrum disorder as well as accurately identified nine out of 10 individuals who did not.

Given the difficulty of recognizing bipolar spectrum disorders pathology and the serious nature of the disorders, this instrument shows promise for use as an accurate screening instrument in clinical practice. The simple dichotomous response and ease of scoring make it applicable to multiple settings. However, further validation and reliability reports are needed to confirm its use in the general population, for primary care, and for research purposes.

CHAPTER 4

Assessment of Addiction and Related Disorders

ADDICTION DISORDERS COMMONLY ENCOUNTERED IN CLINICAL PRACTICE

The category "addiction and related disorders" encompasses a broad range of pathology in the most recent edition of the *Diagnostic and Statistical Manual of Mental Disorders* (*DSM-5*; APA, 2013). Disorders classified under this heading include alcohol-related disorders, caffeine-related disorders, cannabis-related disorders, hallucinogen-related disorders, inhalant-related disorders, opioid-related disorders, sedative/hypnotic-related disorders, stimulant-related disorders, tobacco-related disorders, unknown substance disorders, gambling disorder, neuro-behavioral disorder associated with prenatal alcohol exposure, and Internet use disorder. The majority of these disorders are broken down into the more specific diagnoses of the specific substance use disorder, intoxication, withdrawal, and substance-induced disorder not elsewhere classified. Because disorders related to alcohol and substance use are the most common, and dangerous to physical and psychological health, they receive primary focus in this section. Internet use disorder will also be highlighted, since it is a new disorder in the *DSM-5*.

Alcohol use disorder is characterized by a problematic pattern of alcohol use which leads to clinically significant impairment or distress (APA, 2013). Within the past year, at least two of the following must have occurred for an individual to warrant a diagnosis of alcohol use disorder: (a) alcohol is frequently consumed in greater amounts or for a longer time period than anticipated; (b) frequent desire or unsuccessful attempts to reduce or control alcohol use; (c) excessive time aimed at obtaining, using, and recovering from use; (d) frequent use causes inability to fulfill obligations; (e) continued use despite interpersonal problems; (f) important roles or activities are reduced or eliminated because of alcohol use; (g) physically dangerous activities while under the influence; (h) continued use despite physical or psychological problem stemming from use; (i) tolerance; (j) withdrawal; or (k) craving. Abuse and dependence have been condensed into a single diagnosis in the *DSM-5*, due to the numerous diagnostic problems encountered by differentiating between the two. Instead, severity is characterized according to criterion counts, in which 2–3 criteria indicates mild substance use disorder, 4–5 criteria indicate moderate substance use disorder, and 6 or more criteria indicate severe substance use disorder.

Various other substance abuse disorders within this category require an individual to meet two of the criteria listed above but for their respective substances. Thus, the diagnostic criteria elucidated above can also be applied to cannabis use disorder, caffeine use disorder, hallucinogen use disorder, opioid use disorder, sedative/hypnotic use disorder, stimulant use disorder, tobacco use disorder, and unknown substance use disorder (APA, 2013). Inhalant use disorder is characterized by the existence of at least two of the same criteria detailed above, with the exception of withdrawal, which is not included for diagnosis of inhalant use disorder. Severity ratings for each of these disorders also mirror the severity ratings enumerated above for alcohol use disorder.

Alcohol use disorders and drug use disorders are some of the most common psychiatric disorders diagnosed in the United States (Stinson et al., 2006). In the past year, 8.5% of adults have had an alcohol use disorder, 2% of adults have had a drug use disorder, and 1.1% have had comorbid alcohol use disorders and drug use disorders (Falk, Yi, & Hiller-Sturmhöfel, 2008; Stinson et al.). The prevalence of alcohol use disorders, drug use disorders, and comorbid disorders was highest among men and those aged 18 to 24 years and declined with increasing age (Falk et al.). Although men and women followed similar patterns of alcohol use, drug use, and co-use, men were significantly more likely to use alcohol only, or both alcohol and drugs, while women were more likely than men to abstain from using alcohol and drugs altogether. The risk of alcohol use disorder onset and persistence was elevated among younger males of minority status and older African-American and Hispanic women (Grant et al., 2012). The highest rates of alcohol use were found among Whites, but Native Americans/Alaskan Natives had the highest rates of drug use, alcohol use disorders, drug use disorders, and comorbid disorders. Asian/Pacific Islander men and Hispanic women have been found to have the lowest rates of alcohol, drug, and co-use. Drug use and drug use disorders were associated with higher levels of alcohol consumption and alcohol use disorders, although this relationship cannot be applied in the opposite direction. Those diagnosed with drug use disorders were also differentiated from those with alcohol use disorders, in that they were more frequently male, young, single, and of a lower socioeconomic status (Stinson et al., 2006).

The comorbidity of lifetime alcohol use disorders and drug use disorders is high, ranging from 20–23% (Falk et al., 2008). However, comorbidity is not limited to the common association between alcohol use disorders and drug use disorders, but includes various other psychiatric disorders as well. Social anxiety disorder diagnoses are correlated with significantly increased rates and severity of alcohol abuse and dependence (Schneier et al., 2010). This association is especially troubling because this population is characterized by low rates of treatment seeking. Also, many clients diagnosed with alcohol use disorders or drug use disorders are comorbid with mood disorders, anxiety disorders, or personality disorders, and these comorbid disorders are among the most common mental health disorders in the United States (Falk et al., 2008; Grant et al., 2006). The need for increased clarity in appropriately screening, assessing, and diagnosing those with dual or multiple diagnoses is pressing, given that this population is at an increased risk for being under-identified, misdiagnosed, and ineffectively treated (Morojele, Saban, & Seedat, 2012).

Treatment for alcohol use disorders, drug use disorders, and comorbid disorders has been shown to be efficacious, but treatment-seeking rates are alarmingly low. Stinson et al. (2006) found that only 6% of those with alcohol use disorders, 16% of those with drug use disorders, and 22% of those with comorbid disorders sought treatment to address their respective disorders. Dawson, Grant, Stinson, Chou et al. (2005) obtained slightly improved, but still markedly low rates, finding that 25.5% of those with alcohol dependence sought treatment. Treatments vary from self-help support groups like Alcoholics Anonymous to formal mental health treatment, and both have been proven equally efficacious over an eight-year period (Parker, Marshall, & Ball, 2008; Timko, Moos, Finney, & Lesar, 2000). Recovery rates are promising, given that after one year only 25% of those previously classified as alcohol dependent still met criteria for an alcohol dependence diagnosis (Dawson, Grant, Stinson, Chou et al., 2005). The remaining 18.2% were abstainers, 27.3% were in partial remission, and the rest were asymptomatic or low risk drinkers.

Researchers are continually gaining knowledge of, and examining the criteria currently recommended for diagnosis of, Internet use disorder in the *DSM-5* (APA, 2013). Presently, the presence of the following criteria have been recommended: (a) preoccupation with online gaming; (b) withdrawal symptoms; (c) tolerance; (d) unable to control online gaming use; (e) continued use despite knowledge of negative psychosocial problems; (f) loss of other interests or hobbies due to use; (g) use as an escape or relief from sadness; (h) attempts to hide magnitude of use from others; and (i) lost job, relationship, or other opportunity because of online gaming use. The rationale and severity of Internet use disorder are still being developed.

Although the previous lack of a consistent, standardized, definition of Internet addiction has limited the collection of prevalence data (Byun et al., 2009; Liu & Potenza, 2007), current estimates indicate that somewhere between 1.5% and 11 % of Internet users meet the criteria for problematic Internet use (Liu & Potenza, 2007; Weinstein & Lejoyeux, 2010). Most recently, researchers found that 4% of U.S. adolescents met the criteria for Internet addiction (Liu, Desai, Krishnan-Sarin, Cavallo, & Potenza, 2011). Problematic Internet use is more common among Asian and Hispanic students (Liu et al., 2011) and males (Kormas, Critselis, Janikian, Kafetzis, & Tsitsika, 2011; Liu & Potenza, 2007). Some have speculated that the higher prevalence rate among males can be attributed to their higher likelihood of engaging in online gaming, gambling, and cybersex, all activities associated with compulsive use (Liu & Potenza, 2007). However, although males actually report more time spent online and missing more important activities as a result of Internet use, girls are more likely to report that their Internet use is excessive (Liu et al., 2011).

Problematic Internet use is correlated with using the Internet for sexual information, interactive game-playing, and socialization (Kormas et al., 2011). Because so much attention has been focused on addiction to online gaming, very little consideration has been given to the potential problematic use of social networking sites such as Facebook. Future researchers should seek to address addiction to social networking sites to rectify the paucity of research in this area. Preliminary research shows that social networking site usage is negatively correlated with academic achievement and relationship problems, problems which overlap with criteria necessary for diagnosis of Internet addiction (Kuss & Griffiths, 2011). Furthermore, multiple factors have been found to be predictive of problematic Internet use, including lack of perseverance, social anxiety, family conflict, recent stressors, and substance use (Weinstein & Lejoyeux, 2010).

Overuse of the Internet is associated with a host of other mental health diagnoses and problems, including depression, anxiety, obsessive-compulsive disorder, attention-deficit/hyperactivity disorder, substance use, conduct problems, aggression, and overall psychosocial maladjustment (Kormas et al., 2011; Liu & Potenza, 2007; Liu et al., 2011; Weinstein & Lejoyeux, 2010).

Given the nascence of this disorder, very few researchers have thus far addressed the treatment of Internet addiction. Among those who have, proposed treatments include the use of support groups, time management techniques, cognitive-behavioral therapy, and family therapy (Liu & Potenza, 2007). Weinstein and Lejoyeux (2010) noted that treatment is currently based on psychosocial treatments, rather than the pharmacological treatment methodologies used to help those with other addictive disorders, such as substance use disorders. They refrained from endorsing any treatment over another due to the current scarcity of evidence in the literature. Screening for Internet use disorder will thus prove necessary and valuable for identifying those plagued by problematic Internet use, in order to gain knowledge about how best to treat this population.

In summary, myriad negative consequences of addictive disorders make screening for these disorders absolutely critical. Given the unlikely propensity of those suffering from alcohol or substance use disorders to seek treatment, and the newness of Internet use disorder, it is imperative that clinicians seek to accurately identify potential cases of these disorders in order to deliver treatment in a timely manner.

Highlights of Free-Access Instruments Used to Identify and Monitor Outcomes

A variety of instruments are available to measure the presence and severity of addiction and related disorders. This section provides summaries of recommended commonly used free-access instruments for the assessment of addiction and related disorders.

Alcohol Use Dependence Identification Test (AUDIT)

The World Health Organization originally developed the Alcohol Use Dependence Identification Test to screen for hazardous drinking, harmful drinking, and alcohol dependence in adults (AUDIT; Saunders, Aasland, Babor, De La Fuente, & Grant, 1993). In the years since, various translated (Berner, Kriston, Bentele, & Harter, 2007) and abbreviated (de Meneses-Gaya, Zuardi, Loureiro, & Crippa, 2009) versions of the AUDIT have been validated, including the AUDIT-3, AUDIT-C, AUDIT-QF, AUDIT-PC, AUDIT-4, FAST, and the Five-Shot. The AUDIT is appropriate for use with both male and female adolescents and adults (Kelly, Donovan, Chung, Bukstein, & Cornelius, 2009; Kokotailo, 2004; Miles, Winstock, & Strang, 2001; Santis, Garmendia, Acuna, Alvarado, & Arteaga, 2009). The AUDIT can be accessed free of charge at http://whqlibdoc.who.int/hq/2001/WHO_MSD_MSB_01.6a.pdf.

The AUDIT is a Level A test, meaning that an advanced degree is not needed for administration, scoring, and interpretation. The AUDIT is a self-report instrument composed of 10 Likert-type items, most of which are scored on a five point scale ranging from "never" to "daily or almost daily" (Saunders et al., 1993). The first three items are designed to assess the amount of alcohol consumption, the following three items target the level of alcohol dependence, and the final four items measure consequences of drinking. The least symptomatic response is scored as a zero, with each successive response receiving one, two, three, or four points. Items nine and 10 only have three response choices, and thus the least symptomatic response is scored as a zero, with each successive response receiving two or four points. The maximum possible score on the AUDIT is 40. Scores ranging from 0 to 7 indicate low risk drinking, scores from 8 to 15 indicate risky, hazardous drinking, scores from 16 to 19 indicate high risk, harmful drinking, and scores in excess of 20 indicate high risk, dependent drinking. Many researchers have recommended the use of lower cut-points to more accurately identify cases of hazardous and dependent drinking in various populations. Cut-off scores of five points in the elderly population (Aalto, Alho, Halme, & Seppä, 2011), six points among women (Boschloo et al., 2010; de Meneses-Gaya et al., 2009; Selin, 2003), and somewhere between three and seven points among adolescents (de Meneses-Gaya et al., 2009; Kelly et al., 2009; Kokotailo, 2004; Santis et al., 2009) allowed researchers to obtain optimal balances between sensitivity and specificity.

Scores on the AUDIT have been reported to be both reliable and valid. Internal consistency coefficients ranging from .76 to .83 have been obtained by researchers studying diverse populations (de Meneses-Gaya et al., 2009; Kelly et al., 2009; Santis et al., 2009; Schmidt & Barry, 1995; Selin, 2003). Test-retest reliability estimates are also reported to be good to excellent among adolescents, adults in primary care settings, and the general population (de Meneses-Gaya et al., 2009; Santis et al., 2009; Selin, 2003). Test-retest reliability is optimal among moderate consumers (Selin, 2003). Selin found evidence of poor reliability among low consumers, but this is likely due to the infrequency with which they consume alcohol.

Various sensitivities and specificities have been reported for the AUDIT. In a meta-analysis, Berner et al. (2007) found that, at a cut-off of eight points, sensitivity estimates ranged from .31 to .89 and specificity estimates ranged from .83 to .96 in primary care settings. Among general hospital patients and college students, sensitivity ranged from .72 to .93 and specificity ranged from .78 to .94, while, among the elderly, sensitivity was slightly reduced, ranging from .55 to .83, and specificity increased to .96. Various researchers have advocated for the use of lower cut-points in order to accurately identify the majority of true positives and true negatives (Aalto et al., 2011; Volk, Steinbauer, Cantor, & Holzer, 1997). Those who have opted to use a cut-point of five or six have obtained sensitivities ranging from .61 to .91 and specificities of .60 to .84 (Aalto et al., 2011; Dawson, Grant, Stinson, & Zhou, 2005; Kelly et al., 2009; Kokotailo, 2004; Schmidt & Barry, 1995). Miles, Winstock, and Strang

(2001) provided additional evidence for the predictive validity of scores on the AUDIT by showing scores on the AUDIT to predict self-reported patterns of consumption and total consequences. Furthermore, various abbreviated versions of the AUDIT, including AUDIT-3, AUDIT-C, AUDIT-QF, AUDIT-PC, AUDIT-4, FAST, and Five-Shot, have been found to have psychometrics which are just as strong as, if not superior to, the original AUDIT (de Meneses-Gaya et al., 2009).

The sole major concern with regard to score validity is found in the controversy regarding the most appropriate factor structure of the AUDIT. The AUDIT was originally constructed as a three factor instrument, designed to measure consumption, dependence, and consequences (Saunders et al., 1993). However, many researchers have found a two-factor model to be more appropriate for interpretation (Doyle, Donovan, & Kivlahan, 2007; Rist, Glöckner-Rist, & Demmel, 2009; Shields, Guttmannova, & Caruso, 2004; von der Pahlen et al., 2008). Doyle et al. noted that, while a three-factor model also fits the data well, alcohol dependence and harmful alcohol use are highly correlated; thus, condensing these two factors into a single factor is more sensible. While it may simplify interpretation of the AUDIT using a single raw score, Doyle et al. indicated that the use of the AUDIT as a one-factor screening instrument with just one cut-off score may be problematic.

The advantages of using the AUDIT are manifold. An important advantage of the AUDIT is that it can be used with both male and female adolescents and adults, and has been validated for use with multicultural populations (Volk, Steinbauer, Cantor, & Holzer, 1997), emergency room populations (Kelly et al., 2009), and primary care and hospital inpatient populations (Berner et al., 2007). This versatility among diverse populations renders the AUDIT a valuable tool for effectively screening many different types of people.

Additionally, use of the AUDIT is efficacious because, by targeting the broad spectrum of harmful drinking, rather than only alcoholics, the AUDIT is able to identify and discriminate among people with varied levels of harmful drinking. This sensitivity to different levels of hazardous drinking sets the AUDIT apart from the CAGE and the MAST, other common screening tests for alcohol problems which focus mainly on dependence, the most severe end of the spectrum (Miles et al., 2001). Although the most recent edition of the DSM will use ratings of severity rather than differentiated levels of harmful, hazardous, and dependent drinking (APA, 2013), the sensitivity of the AUDIT will likely remain useful. The superiority of the AUDIT is further supported by the findings of other researchers that the AUDIT outperforms numerous other measures of addiction, including the RAPS4-QF, the RUFT-Cut, the CAGE, and the CRAFFT (de Meneses-Gaya et al., 2009; Kelly et al., 2009). Especially notable is the superiority of the AUDIT compared to the CAGE and CRAFFT when used with adolescents.

Furthermore, the emphasis of the AUDIT on hazardous consumption rather than a narrow focus on adverse consequences also serves to identify those clients who may not yet be experiencing problems as a result of their drinking, but are at risk for developing such problems. It is likely for this reason that the first three questions of the AUDIT, the consumption items, are increasingly being used to identify risky drinking (Dawson, Grant, Stinson, Chou et al., 2005).

The only notable disadvantages of the AUDIT are the administration time and the fact that it is unable to screen for the risky use of substances other than alcohol. Finally, the propensity of the AUDIT to focus on current, rather than lifetime, drinking could be viewed as either an advantage or a disadvantage. For instance, the current focus would help pinpoint risky drinking in the immediate present and future, but could overlook problematic drinking in the past which could be predictive of future problems.

In conclusion, the AUDIT is a useful screening instrument for detecting harmful and dependent drinking among male and female adolescents and adults. Due to its efficiency and psychometric rigor in both its full and abbreviated versions, the AUDIT provides an optimal balance of psychometric strength and clinical utility. Clinicians are encouraged to consider lower cut-points for women, adolescents, and the elderly, in order to maximize the potential for identifying cases of risky or dependent drinking. The AUDIT is highly recommended for use in school and university settings in order to identify problematic patterns of consumption and resulting consequences as early as possible.

Alcohol, Smoking, and Substance Involvement Screening Test (ASSIST)

The World Health Organization developed the Alcohol, Smoking, and Substance Involvement Screening Test (ASSIST) to screen for psychoactive substance use and related problems (Ali et al., 2002). The most recent version, the ASSIST Version 3.0, has been translated for use in Chinese, Hindi, Spanish, Arabic, Farsi, French, German, and Portuguese, and is available free of charge at http://www.who.int/substance_abuse/activities/assist_test/en/index.html. Originally developed for adults in primary care, the ASSIST is appropriate for use with adolescents and adults in primary health care, drug treatment facilities, and mental health settings (Hides et al., 2009; Humeniuk et al., 2008; Newcombe, Humeniuk, & Ali, 2005; Spear et al., 2009), and some believe the ASSIST would be useful in identifying at-risk individuals in the general population, such as in schools or general public health settings (Davis, Thomas, Jesseman, & Mazan, 2009; Humeniuk et al., 2008).

The ASSIST is an interviewer-directed questionnaire that requires approximately 15 to 20 minutes for administration. Prior to beginning the interview, respondents are provided with a response card, which lists the substances they will be asked about and the required response choices for each question (Ali et al., 2002). Question one dichotomously assesses lifetime use of the following substances: tobacco products, alcoholic beverages, cannabis, cocaine, amphetamines, inhalants, sedatives, hallucinogens, opiods, and other. Questions two through seven are asked separately for each substance the respondent indicated ever having used. For questions two through five, responses are assessed using a five-point Likert scale ranging from "never" to "daily or almost daily." For questions six through eight, interviewees must choose one of three responses of increasing frequency: "no, never," "yes, but not in the past three months," or "yes, in the past three months." Taken as a whole, the ASSIST seeks to identify dependence and consequences of problematic substance use and evaluate potential risk.

Interviewers total the raw score points obtained in items two through seven for each substance to calculate Specific Substance Involvement (SSI) scores (Ali et al., 2002). A Total Substance Involvement (TSI) score can also be obtained by summing all points, but SSI scores are more valuable when interpreting results. A score ranging from zero to three for any of the substances presents a low risk and no further action. For all substances except alcohol, a score between four and 26 indicates moderate risk and a need for brief intervention. Interviewees must score between an 11 and 26 for alcohol to warrant brief intervention and a moderate risk status. If a respondent receives a score in excess of 26 for any of the substances, the respondent is classified as high risk and dependent, and more intensive treatment is recommended. There is minor disagreement in the literature regarding the most appropriate cut-points for adolescent use of alcohol, cannabis, and amphetamines (Davis et al., 2009; Hides et al., 2009); thus, it seems that researchers may need to lower cut-points for adolescents as they learn more about the usefulness of the ASSIST among this population. Brief cards are provided with the ASSIST which list the physical, emotional, interpersonal, and psychological problems associated with excessive use of each substance, as well as the dangers associated with injecting (Ali et al., 2002).

Ample evidence exists to support the reliability and validity of scores on the ASSIST. Ali et al. (2002) found test-retest reliability coefficients ranging from .58 to .90 for individual items, with most reliabilities categorized as either good or excellent. Multiple researchers reported internal consistency coefficients of .89 and above for TSI scores, and .65 and above for SSI scores, with most SSI scores in the high .80s (Hides et al., 2009; Humeniuk et al., 2008). Sensitivities ranging from .78 to .91 and specificities ranging from .64 to .82 have been reported for the overall measure, and all sensitivity and specificity values for specific substances exceeded .58, with most in the .70s and .80s (Hides et al.; Newcombe et al., 2005).

There is an abundance of evidence to support the concurrent, construct, discriminative, and predictive validity of ASSIST scores. Concurrent validity is evidenced by the fact that those with a current DSM diagnosis of either substance abuse or dependence achieved significantly higher TSI scores than those without a diagnosis (Hides et al., 2009; Newcombe et al., 2005). SSI scores for cannabis, alcohol, amphetamines, and opiates were also significantly higher for individuals with these disorders. Additionally, self-reported use of substances, as measured by the ASSIST, were significantly correlated with the presence of these substances in hair samples (Humeniuk et al., 2008). Concurrent validity is further evidenced by multiple significant correlations with various measures of addiction, including the Addiction Severity Index—Lite (ASI-Lite; r = .76–.88), the Severity of Dependence Scale (SDS; r = .59–.67), the AUDIT (r = .82–.84), and the Revised Fagerstrom Tolerance Questionnaire (RFTQ; r = .78) (Humeniuk et al., 2008; Newcombe et al., 2005). The ASSIST TSI score is also significantly correlated with the Maudsley Addiction Profile, a general measure of physical and psychological health (MAP; r = .57; Humeniuk et al., 2008), providing further evidence of construct validity. Furthermore, the ASSIST is able to effectively discriminate between low risk and abuse groups as well as between abuse and dependence groups when using TSI scores or SSI scores for alcohol, cannabis, cocaine, or amphetamines (Humeniuk et al., 2008; Newcombe et al., 2005). Predictive validity is showcased by the similarity of ASSIST scores obtained at baseline and follow-up (Newcombe et al., 2005). Currently, investigation into the factor structure of the ASSIST is lacking.

The advantages of the ASSIST certainly seem to outweigh its disadvantages. The interviewer-led format of the ASSIST allows interviewers to build a rapport with respondents and probe for further information. Although lengthier than most screening instruments, the ASSIST provides a comprehensive screening of all substances which people could be abusing, and allows interviewers to pinpoint dependence and consequences due to overall substance abuse or specific substance abuse. The ASSIST is able to discriminate among non-problematic drug use, drug abuse, and dependence, but discriminates most effectively between low risk and moderate risk use (Newcombe et al., 2005). Efficaciousness in discriminating between low risk and moderate risk groups is optimal for screening, but would render the ASSIST less useful when discriminating between levels of moderate and high severity. Also, the cards provided, which list the risks associated with repeated excessive use of each substance, could be especially beneficial for school personnel or other service providers with minimal training in the effects of various substances. The information provided on these cards could ensure that the interviewer possesses adequate knowledge of the subject and is able to share that knowledge with those in need. Finally, there is strong evidential support for the reliability and validity of scores obtained on the ASSIST, but research into its factor structure is warranted.

Overall, the ASSIST is a well-researched and psychometrically sound instrument appropriate for screening for psychoactive substance use and related problems in male and female adolescent and adult populations. Although it has mainly been used with primary care and drug treatment facility populations, many researchers believe that the ASSIST would be useful and appropriate for screening in the general population (Davis et al., 2009; Humeniuk et al., 2008). Future research should focus on the possibility of differential cut-points for substance abuse and dependence among adolescents. The ASSIST is therefore recommended as providing an excellent comprehensive measure of non-problematic use, abuse, and dependence for various substances.

CRAFFT

Developed by the Center for Adolescent Substance Abuse Research (CeASAR, 2009), the CRAFFT is a mnemonic screening device designed specifically for use with adolescents between the ages of 14 and 21 years. The CRAFFT is a brief screen for alcohol and other substance abuse disorders. The CRAFFT is available in English, Chinese, Haitian Creole, French, Hebrew, Japanese, Khmer, Laotian, Russian, Portuguese, Spanish, Turkish, and Vietnamese. The CRAFFT is intended for use as an interviewer-directed screening instrument, but a self-administered questionnaire format is also available. Both formats can be found, free of charge, at http://www.ceasar-boston.org/clinicians/crafft.php

The CRAFFT is a Level B test, designed to be used by a professional clinician in the mental health field (CaESAR, 2009). The CRAFFT is divided into two parts. In Part A, respondents are asked to respond affirmatively or negatively to three questions which assess alcohol use, marijuana use, and other substance use in the past year. If a respondent answers negatively to all three questions in Part A, he is only required to respond to the first item in Part B. Respondents who answer affirmatively to any of the three questions in Part A are required to respond to all six items in Part B. Part B is composed of six yes or no questions in which the key words spell the mnemonic CRAFFT (Car, Relax, Alone, Forget, Family or Friends, Trouble). Each "yes" response in Part B is worth one point. A score of two or higher classifies the respondent as high-risk and indicates a need for additional assessment.

The reliability and validity of scores on the CRAFFT have been supported by various researchers. Levy et al. (2004) reported an intraclass correlation coefficient of .93 and found that kappa coefficients for individual items ranged from .31 to .86. While the CRAFFT can be administered as a lifetime or past-year screen, Levy et al. found the past-year version to be the most reliable. Coefficient alphas of .73 to .81 indicate that internal consistency estimates are mostly adequate for screening purposes (Cummins et al., 2003; Subramaniam, Cheok, Verma, Wong, & Chong, 2010). Concurrent validity is supported by the finding that users of prescription opiods for non-medical reasons are more likely than non-users to screen positively on the CRAFFT (McCabe et al., 2012). The strong correlation found between diagnostic classifications for substance use and dependence and CRAFFT scores further supports the concurrent validity of the instrument (Knight, Sherritt, Shrier, Harris, & Chang, 2002). Furthermore, Cummins et al. (2003) found that the CRAFFT effectively identified all frequent users of alcohol and marijuana. Sensitivity and specificity levels of the CRAFFT mirror those of the AUDIT, the gold standard of screening for alcohol problems. Sensitivity estimates have been found to range from .76 to .92, while specificity estimates range from .64 to .94 (Cummins et al.; Knight et al., 2002; Knight, Sherritt, Harris, Gates, & Chang, 2003). The sensitivity and specificity estimates of CRAFFT scores are similar for identifying any problem, disorder, and dependence (Knight et al. 2002), rendering the CRAFFT ideally suited to detect varying levels of problematic alcohol or other substance use and dependence.

There are various advantages and disadvantages of the CRAFFT. The most important advantage is the brevity of the screening questionnaire. The CRAFFT is ideally suited for both efficient and effective screening for alcohol and other substance abuse problems, including recreational use of prescription drugs (McCabe et al., 2012). This combination of brevity and the ability to identify numerous levels of problematic substance abuse prior to dependence is impressive. Furthermore, the CRAFFT has been validated for use with various racial and ethnic minority groups, making the CRAFFT a valuable and appropriate screening tool for multicultural populations (Cummins et al., 2003; Knight et al., 2002). Recent research has indicated the utility of the CRAFFT in assessing pregnant young adults to reduce harmful outcomes from prenatal alcohol exposure as well (Braaten, Briegleb, Hauke, Niamkey, & Chang, 2008). Given the findings of Knight et al. (2007) that adolescents prefer answering substance abuse questions via paper and pencil questionnaires rather than through interview formats, the CRAFFT is especially valuable because it can be administered in both formats. This versatility enhances the applicability of the CRAFFT in various situations and allows clinicians to administer screening via the best possible method for each individual client.

The only notable disadvantage of the CRAFFT is the fact that it is in need of additional score reliability and validity evidence. Although evidence thus far has been overwhelmingly positive, the lack of research found in the literature regarding this decade-old instrument was surprising. Additional inquiry into the factor structure and concurrent validity of the CRAFFT is warranted. Furthermore, some disagreement currently exists regarding whether the optimal cut-point of the CRAFFT is a raw score of one (Knight et al., 2003, Subramaniam et al., 2010) or two (Cummins et al., 2003; Knight et al., 2002), with some even suggesting that a cut-point of three is essential for identifying frequent use of other drugs (Cummins et al., 2003).

The CRAFFT is thus highly recommended as a brief and effective screen for problematic alcohol and other substance use among adolescents. While additional evidence of reliability and validity would be useful, the extant literature supports the use of the CRAFFT with multicultural adolescent populations. Its strengths lie in its conciseness and ability to identify problematic drinking or substance use behaviors prior to dependence.

ONLINE COGNITION SCALE (OCS)

The Online Cognition Scale was one of the first instruments developed to assess Internet addiction (OCS; Davis, Flett, & Besser, 2002). Also sometimes referred to as the Davis Online Cognition Scale (DOCS), the OCS has been translated into Turkish and Chinese, and Jia and Jia (2009) recently developed an abbreviated version. The OCS is appropriate for use with male and female adolescents and adults. Now one of the most widely used self-report inventories of Internet addiction, it can be accessed for free at http://www.ndsec.org/2010connectionhandouts/Addressing%20

Mental%20Health%20Issues%20in%20Schools%20Using%20Cognitive%20Behavior%20Therapy/OCS.pdf.

The OCS is a Level A test, meaning that advanced training is not required for administration and interpretation. The OCS can be administered either individually or in groups, and takes approximately 15 minutes to complete. The OCS is composed of 36 items that assess cognitions related to Internet use on a seven-point Likert-type scale, ranging from "strongly disagree" to "strongly agree" (Davis et al., 2002). Taken together, these 36 items represent the four domains of loneliness/depression, social comfort, distraction, and impulse control. Item 12 is reverse scored and then all items are summed to obtain a total score. The items which correspond to each of the four dimensions are also identified in order to provide scorers with the option of calculating subscale scores. The original authors failed to provide guidelines for score interpretation, but subsequent researchers have identified that scores in excess of 78 for females and 92 for males indicate problematic Internet usage (Özcan & Buzlu, 2007). Test administrators should take into consideration that scores just below this threshold likely indicate that respondents are at an elevated risk for developing cognitions and behaviors associated with problematic Internet usage.

The reliability and validity of scores on the OCS have received ample support. Özcan and Buzlu (2005) reported test-retest reliability coefficients of .90 for the total scale and .76–.89 for the various subscales. Internal consistency coefficients for the scale as a whole have all been reported to exceed .85, while internal consistency coefficients for each of the subscales ranged from .77 to .87 in both the full and abbreviated versions (Davis et al., 2002; Jia & Jia, 2009; Özcan & Buzlu). Davis et al. (2002) constructed the OCS based on an extensive literature search of the most important dimensions of problematic Internet use and also adapted items from related measures of procrastination, depression, impulsivity, and pathological gambling, all either part of, or very similar to, the construct of Internet addiction. These methods of item construction lend support to the content validity of the OCS.

Evidence in support of the construct validity of scores on the OCS is abundant. The confirmatory factor analysis originally used by Davis et al. (2002) yielded four factors: loneliness/depression, social comfort, distraction, and diminished impulse control. Jia and Jia (2009) confirmed the satisfactory fit of the four-factor model. However, because scores on loneliness/depression, social comfort, and diminished impulse control were highly correlated, Jia and Jia collapsed these three factors into a single factor, labeled dependency. The resulting two-factor model also demonstrated a good fit and served to increase efficiency, since items from the three related factors were condensed to allow for a more even distribution of items among factors.

Scores on the OCS are positively correlated with measures of both depression (r = .34) and loneliness (r = .34) and negatively correlated with perceived social support (r = -.32) (Özcan & Buzlu, 2005, 2007). Scores on each of the four subscales are correlated with number of hours spent online per week, as well as various measures of rejection sensitivity, procrastination, loneliness/depression, and scores on the Internet Behavior and Attitude Scale (IBAS), which also assesses problematic Internet use (Davis et al., 2002; Nalwa & Anand, 2003). Global scores on the OCS are also highly correlated (r = .70) with total scores on the Compulsive Internet Use Scale (CIUS) (Meerkerk, van der Eijnden, Vermulst, & Garretsen, 2009). In addition to this evidence of convergent validity, concurrent validity of scores on the OCS was demonstrated by the fact that those participants classified as dependent on the Internet scored significantly higher than participants classified as non-dependent on the OCS (Nalwa & Anand, 2003). Higher scores on the OCS are also associated with increased amounts of online interactive and entertainment activities among both adolescents and adults, and increased visits to adult websites among adults (Davis et al., 2002; Jia & Jia, 2009; Özcan & Buzlu, 2007).

Thus, there are various advantages and disadvantages to assessing problematic Internet use with the OCS. First, the OCS is useful both as a clinical assessment of Internet addiction and as a screening measure that could prove valuable in predicting inappropriate Internet usage in a variety of settings, given that Davis et al. (2002) found that OCS scores predicted being disciplined for inappropriate Internet usage at school or work. Also, the evidence in support of the score reliability and validity of both the 10- and 36-item versions allows the administrator to choose an equitable alternative in the interest of time. Finally, most screening tests for problematic Internet usage focus solely on adolescents, so the validation of the OCS with adults extends its applicability and makes it quite valuable (Jia & Jia, 2009).

As clinicians continue to accumulate the diagnostic criteria for Internet addiction, researchers are tasked with the job of establishing predictive validity. Also, given that the OCS was developed in 2002, researchers may need to verify that the constructs perceived to underlie problematic Internet usage a decade ago still remain relevant with the many changes and differences in Internet usage today. Finally, future researchers should focus on determining appropriate cut-points to aid in score interpretation.

The robust psychometrics of the OCS substantiates its wide use in both research and clinical applications. Although additional evidence of its continued score reliability and validity are needed as the Internet continues to evolve, the OCS is the best assessment of problematic Internet usage currently available for free access. The OCS is thus recommended for use in the screening and assessment of Internet addiction with adolescents and adults.

Chapter 5

Assessment of AD/HD, Disruptive, Impulse Control, Obsessive Compulsive and Related Disorders

Attention deficit/hyperactivity disorder (AD/HD), disruptive behavior disorders, impulse control, obsessive compulsive and related disorders are commonly experienced by children, adolescents, and adults, and cause significant impairments in life functioning. The most recent edition of the *DSM-5* (APA, 2013) has integrated disruptive, impulse control, and conduct disorders, including oppositional defiant, intermittent explosive, conduct, and unspecified or otherwise specified disruptive or impulse control disorders. AD/HD is now categorized as a neurodevelopmental disorder, rather than a disruptive behavior; however, inattentive and/or hyperactive type will be covered in this chapter. The obsessive compulsive and related disorders category includes obsessive compulsive, body dysmorphic, hoarding, hair-pulling (trichotillomania), skin-picking, substance-induced obsessive-compulsive or related disorders, and obsessive-compulsive or related disorders attributable to another medical condition or not elsewhere classified. This chapter will focus primarily on AD/HD, disruptive, impulse control, and obsessive compulsive and related disorders.

ATTENTION DEFICIT/HYPERACTIVITY DISORDER (AD/HD)

Attention deficit/hyperactivity disorder (AD/HD) is characterized by a consistent display of behavior and cognitive functioning that causes substantial disturbances in social, educational, or work environments (APA, 2013). Individuals must display six or more inattentive and/or hyperactive/impulsive symptoms for six months to qualify for diagnosis. For adolescents and adults, four or more symptoms must be present. Combined presentation may be diagnosed if an individual meets criteria for both inattention and hyperactivity symptoms. Other specified AD/HD may be possible if the criterion is not met for either.

Inattention symptoms include: (1) lacks consideration to detail or makes thoughtless errors; (2) trouble focusing on tasks; (3) appears not to pay attention when spoken to; (4) often fails to follow directions or complete tasks; (5) trouble organizing and managing time/tasks; (6) evades or is unwilling to perform responsibilities that necessitate continuous mental exertion; (7) misplaces essential materials for school or work; (8) easily diverted by internal thoughts or external sounds; and (9) careless in everyday procedures (APA, 2013). Predominately inattentive presentation is diagnosed if the individual meets inattention criteria and fails to meet hyperactive criteria even when displaying at least three of the symptoms. Inattentive presentation is diagnosed if the individual displays no more than two hyperactive symptoms.

Hyperactivity/impulsivity symptoms include: (1) moves hands/feet restlessly or body about in his or her seat; (2) vacates his or her seat when s/he should be seated; (3) plays around excessively in inappropriate situations; (4) participates in leisure activities in an unusually loud manner; (5) unable to remain stagnant for a prolonged time period; (6) extraordinarily garrulous; (7) exclaims an answer before a query is finished; (8) impatient; and (9) disrupts others' tasks or conversations (APA, 2013). Predominately hyperactive/impulsive presentation is diagnosed if the individual meets hyperactive criteria and fails to meet inattention criteria.

For diagnosis, the inattention and/or hyperactive/impulsive symptoms must have been present before the age of 12 years (APA, 2013). The symptoms must be present in two or more settings and cause significant interference with social, occupational, or educational functioning. In addition, the symptoms must not be best explained by another mental disorder.

AD/HD prevalence estimates for children and adolescents often vary based on survey methodology. In 2003, the National Survey of Children's Health (NSCH) estimated the prevalence rate for children aged 4 to 17 years was 7.8% (Centers for Disease Control and Prevention (CDC), 2005). Results indicated that 4.4 million children had been diagnosed with AD/HD and 56% of those reported taking medication for the disorder. Disparities between gender, age, and race were reported with more white or black non-Hispanic teenage males diagnosed with AD/HD. Other risk factors for increased hyperactive or behavior difficulties include single-parent homes and low-income families (Strine et al., 2006).

AD/HD is often comorbid with other behavioral problems. Children with a history of AD/HD are more likely to experience emotional issues, peer relation difficulties, and conduct problems (Strine et al., 2006). Children with AD/HD are more likely to encounter learning difficulties (Pastor & Reuben, 2008). Children with AD/HD are also more likely to experience major injuries that require hospital care than children without AD/HD (Leibson, Katusic, Barbaresi, Ransom & O'Brien., 2001). These functioning impairments may have a significant effect on children's educational achievement as well as general health and well-being.

Adult AD/HD has recently gained the attention of mental health professionals, as it was originally thought to occur only in children and adolescents. Adult AD/HD prevalence is estimated at 4.4% in the general population with 2.6% meeting full criteria in childhood (Kessler, Adler et al., 2006). Adult AD/HD is often comorbid with mood, anxiety, substance, or intermittent explosive disorder, and is correlated with unemployment and previous marriage. Adults with AD/HD also report significant issues with self-care, mobility, and cognition. Despite these difficulties, only 25.2% of adults report receiving treatment for AD/HD. Early identification and treatment of AD/HD is recommended to prevent long-term negative impact on functioning in children and adults. Thus, it is important for clinicians, parents, and educators alike to be able to identify AD/HD symptoms for early intervention.

Disruptive & Impulse Control Disorders

Oppositional defiant disorder (ODD) is characterized by a pattern of consistent bad-tempered mood with rebellious behavior. The individual must display four or more of the eight symptoms from any of the three categories with one or more people. The first category, "angry/irritable mood," contains the following behaviors: (1) reacts with rage easily; (2) is easily perturbed by others; and (3) is irate or bitter. The second category, "argumentative/defiant behavior," contains the following: (4) argues with adults; (5) blatantly defies authority; (6) purposely annoys others; and (7) blames others for their wrongdoing. The last category, "vindictiveness," is described as (8) has been malicious at least two times in the past six months (APA, 2013). For children under five years of age, the behavior must occur on most days for six months, whereas, for children older than five years, the behavior must occur once a week for six months. The behavior must significantly affect social, educational, or vocational functioning and may occur in one or more settings.

Conduct disorder (CD) is characterized by persistent behavior which infringes on the rights of others or violates societal norms with the presence of three or more of the 15 behaviors in the past year from any category and one behavior in the past six months. The first category includes "aggression to people or animals": (1) threatens others; (2) instigates physical fights; (3) has used a weapon that can inflict severe injury on others; (4) has been physically brutal to people; (5) has been physically malicious to animals; (6) has physically confronted and robbed a victim; or (7) has used force to engage others in carnal actions. The second category includes "destruction of property": (8) purposeful fire-setting to cause significant destruction; or (9) purposeful destruction of others' property. The third category includes "deceitfulness or theft": (10) has engaged in breaking and entering into another's property; (11) scams others; or (12) pilfered items without conflict. The last category includes "serious violations of rules": (13) stays out past parental restrictions prior to age 13 years; (14) has run away from parental or guardian home overnight more than twice, or once for a prolonged period of time; or (15) frequent absentee from school prior to age 13 years (APA, 2013).

These behaviors must cause significant impairment in social, educational, or occupational functioning. If the individual is 18 years or older, the criteria for antisocial personality disorder must not be met (APA, 2013). Types of conduct disorder are related to age of onset. Behaviors present prior to age 10 years are labeled childhood-onset type; absence of behaviors prior to age 10 years is labeled adolescent-onset type; and unknown age of onset is labeled unspecified-onset type. Severity of the disorder should be specified as mild, moderate, or severe, based on number of conduct problems and level of harm to others.

A proposed addition to the *DSM-5* is a callous and unemotional specifier for conduct disorder (APA, 2013). These individuals must meet criteria for conduct disorder and show two or more of the following behaviors in more than one interaction or setting for at least a year: (1) absence of regret; (2) indifference to others' feelings; (3) uninterested in achievement in education or occupation; or (4) dearth of affect. Other specified and unspecified disruptive or impulse control disorders may be diagnosed if the individual does not meet specific criteria, yet displays a significant impairment.

Symptoms of ODD and CD have a high degree of overlap (Maughan, Rowe, Messer, Goodman, & Meltzer, 2004). A diagnosis of ODD may often preclude a diagnosis of CD. In a nationally representative sample, researchers found that 62% of boys and 56% of girls with CD also met the criteria for ODD. Comorbidity with other non-antisocial DSM diagnoses is highly likely for children and adolescents with a history of ODD or CD. The study found that 46% of boys and 36% of girls with ODD and 46% of boys and 39% of girls with CD met criteria for at least one non-antisocial disorder. The most common comorbid disorders included anxiety and depressive disorders and AD/HD.

Prevalence estimates of ODD and CD are higher for boys. One study found that 2.1% of boys and less than 1% of girls met criteria for CD, while 3.2% of boys and 1.4% of girls met criteria for ODD (Maughan et al., 2004). Researchers noted a significant difference between teacher and parent ratings, with teachers indicating a greater number of symptoms in boys. Prevalence rates for ODD tend to decrease with age, while CD prevalence rates increase through adolescence.

Conduct disorder can cause significant disturbances to a child's or adolescent's functioning that can follow into adulthood. Researchers found that adults with a previous history of CD were more likely to have comorbid psychiatric diagnoses (Morcillo et al., 2012). Common *DSM* diagnoses reported for men and women included a variety of externalizing disorders such as substance abuse, bipolar, and histrionic personality disorders. Women were more likely than men to be diagnosed with substance abuse disorders, while men were more likely to be diagnosed with AD/HD and obsessive-compulsive disorder. Researchers also found that the likelihood for an adult psychiatric disorder increased as the number of CD symptoms exhibited increased.

Intermittent explosive disorder is characterized by an individual who is unable to control his or her aggression, which results in impulsive destructive episodes (APA, 2013). Previous national sample occurrence estimates revealed high rates at 7.3% for lifetime and 3.9% for twelve-month prevalence (Kessler, Cocarro et al., 2006). However, previous *DSM-IV-TR* criteria included those under 18 years, while *DSM-5* criteria states that the individual must be at least 18 years of age (APA, 2013). In order to meet criteria for the disorder, the episode must result in either (a) physical or verbal belligerence toward people, animals, or property, on an average of two times weekly in the last three months; or (b) three extreme episodes that lead to physical assault toward a person or destruction of property over the past year, with one episode occurring in the last three months. The episode must also be extremely out of proportion to the activating stressor, not planned, not best explained by another mental disorder, substance, or general medical condition, and must cause significant life function impairment.

Obsessive Compulsive and Related Disorders

Obsessive Compulsive Disorder may include the presence of obsessions, compulsions, or both occurring together. Incidence among U.S. adults is estimated at 1% for twelve-month prevalence (Kessler, Chiu, Demler, & Walters, 2005). An obsession involves the relentless preoccupation with obtrusive thoughts or urges that cause significant agitation (APA, 2013). To qualify as an obsession, the individual must attempt to resist the thoughts or urges or reduces them through performing a compulsion. A compulsion involves repeated physical or psychological actions which one feels forced to complete in response to their obsessions. The compulsions must be completed to minimize distress or to thwart a precipitating event, which in reality, has no connection with the action. In addition, the obsessions and/or compulsions must be onerous; cause impairment to an individual's functioning, and cannot be better attributed to another substance, medical condition, or *DSM-5* disorder. Clinicians should indicate whether the individual has good/fair, poor, or absent insight related to the validity of their beliefs.

Body dysmorphic disorder is characterized by an individual's fixation with perceptual imperfections in their physical appearance which are unobservable or only minor to others (APA, 2013). Prevalence rates are estimated at 2.4% in the U.S. adult population with similar rates for males and females (Koran, Abujaoude, Large, & Serpe, 2008). During the development of the disorder, the individual also must have engaged in recurrent physical (i.e., looking in the mirror) or mental (i.e., comparing themselves with others) actions. The symptoms must cause substantial tension or impairment in daily functioning, is not best accounted for by another medical disorder or eating disorder (APA, 2013). A clinician may classify the disorder as muscle dysmorphia in which the individual perceives their muscular build to be deficient. Clinicians should indicate whether the individual has good/fair, poor, or absent insight into the beliefs of their appearance.

Hoarding is characterized by an individual's inability to throw away personal belongings regardless of their monetary value (APA, 2013). The individual feels an apparent need to save the items and experiences substantial angst connected with parting from the belongings. The extreme buildup of possessions renders living areas inaccessible and any clean areas are only possible due to an intervention. Little is known about the pervasiveness of the disorder as it was previously considered a feature of obsessive-compulsive disorder. The hoarding must cause significant anxiety and impairment to the individual's functioning including the inability to sustain a safe household. The symptoms must occur in absence from another medical or psychiatric disorder. A feature of the disorder is excessive acquisition, in which the individual goes through great lengths to gather, purchase, or steal unnecessary items. Clinicians should indicate whether the individual has good/fair, poor, or absent insight into the problematic nature of their behaviors.

Hair pulling, also referred to as trichotillomania, is characterized by frequent hair pulling which results in loss of hair (APA, 2013). The individual must have had failed attempts to minimize or put an end to the hair pulling. The hair pulling causes the individual significant stress or impairment in social or occupational functioning. The hair pulling must not be best accounted for by another medical or *DSM-5* condition. Skin picking disorder is a new proposed disorder in the *DSM-5*. This disorder is characterized by excessive skin picking that leads to abrasions and attempts to minimize or end the picking have failed. The skin picking causes the individual significant stress or impairment in daily functioning. The disorder must not be best accounted for by the consumption of a substance, a medical condition, or another *DSM-5* disorder.

Given the pervasiveness and potential long-term effects of the aforementioned disorders on mental health and educational, occupational, or social functioning an early diagnosis and intervention is necessary. Proper treatment can prevent significant life impairments. Thus, health professionals, parents, and educators need to become aware of reliable assessment tools to identify these disorders for further treatment and monitoring.

Highlights of Free-Access Instruments Used to Identify and Monitor Outcomes

There are several assessment tools available to assess the presence and severity of AD/HD, disruptive and impulse control disorders and obsessive compulsive disorders. This section will highlight some of the most commonly used free-access instruments for self, clinician, or parent/teacher use. Currently, there is a lack of validated free-access instruments to assess oppositional defiant, intermittent explosive, body dysmorphic, hair-pulling, and skin-picking disorders.

WHO Adult AD/HD Self-Report Scale

The World Health Organization (WHO) and the Workgroup on Adult AD/HD, which included researchers from New York University Medical School and Harvard Medical School, developed the WHO Adult AD/HD Self-Report Scale (ASRS). The scale was designed to assess symptomology of AD/HD in adults. The instrument has been revised several times, with the most recent version (at the time of writing) referred to as the ASRS version 1.1. The instrument has also been translated and validated in both Spanish and Chinese populations (Ramos-Quiroga et al., 2009; Yeh, Gau, Kessler, & Wu, 2008). It can be accessed, for free, online at http://www.addcoach4u.com/adultaddtest.html.

The original ASRS is an 18-item self-report instrument that contains nine items related to inattentive behaviors and nine items related to hyperactivity/impulsivity (Kessler, Chiu et al., 2005). The instrument should be clinician administered as a screening tool and positive screens should be followed up by a clinical interview. Clients rank the frequency of the symptom experienced during the past six months on a five-point scale from 0–4: never (0), rarely (1), sometimes (2), often (3), and very often (4). Responses of often or very often are considered clinically significant symptoms for 11 items. Responses of sometimes, often, or very often are considered clinically significant for seven items. Items are summed for a total score. Scores may range from 0–72. Positive screening follows *DSM-IV* criteria, which recommends six or more significant symptoms for diagnosis.

Scores on the 18-item ASRS have been reported as valid and reliable. Internal consistency has been reported at .88 (Adler et al., 2006). The ASRS demonstrates high concurrent validity with a rater-administrated version of the scale. Kessler, Chiu et al. (2005) found an unweighted six-item screener outperformed the weighted 18-item instrument in specificity and sensitivity. Kessler et al. (2007) reported psychometric properties of the six-item screener to have moderate internal consistency ranging from .63 to .72 and test-retest reliability ranging from .58 to .77. Kessler et al. (2007) recommended the six-item version for initial screening and finding of AD/HD cases, as it is simple and can be completed in less than two minutes.

Based on these findings, the instrument was revised and divided into two separate sections. Part A contains the six questions that were found to be most predictive of an AD/HD diagnosis and Part B contains the remaining 12 questions, which are most closely related to impairment (http://www.addcoach4u.com/adultaddtest.html). This instrument is referred to as the ASRS version 1.1. Clients are asked whether they never, rarely, sometimes, often, or very often experience a symptom. Clients place a checkmark in the corresponding column. In Part A, for items 1–3, an indication of sometimes, often, or very often is considered clinically significant. For items 4–6, an indication of often or very often is considered clinically significant. If four or more items are considered clinically significant, the clinician is instructed to move forward with a clinical interview for diagnosis. The remaining items in Part B help the clinician to gain insight into the frequency or severity of functional impairments for possible diagnosis.

The ASRS is valuable as a screening tool to identify adults with AD/HD. The brevity and simplicity of the instrument renders it useful for a variety of clients and settings. While the instrument is widely used, a disadvantage is the lack of published psychometric data. Further research is needed to validate the ASRS version 1.1 for use in the general population. As the ASRS evaluates the frequency of symptoms, information obtained from the ASRS can also be useful in evaluating treatment effectiveness.

Wender Utah Rating Scale

The Wender Utah Rating Scale (WURS) was designed to measure adults' retrospective perception of their childhood AD/HD (Mackin & Horner, 2005). As a constituent for *DSM* diagnosis for adult AD/HD is its presence in childhood, this instrument seeks to assess the significance of pathology as a child. The WURS has been translated in multiple languages and used in a variety of populations. Two versions of the WURS exist, the WURS-61 and the WURS-25. It can be accessed, for free, online at http://www.venturafamilymed.org/Documents/Wender_Utah%20Rating%20Scale.pdf.

The original WURS instrument contains 61 items pertaining to the client's memory of his or her childhood behavior (Mackin & Horner, 2005). Respondents are asked to rate the frequency of the behavior on a five point scale from 0 to 4: not at all/very slightly (0); mildly (1); moderately (2); quite a bit (3); and very much (4). Twenty-five of the items are related to DSM criteria and are used to differentiate between those with or without AD/HD for diagnosis. The 25 items are summed for a total score. Scores may range from 0 to 100. A cut-off score of 46 or above is recommended for a positive AD/HD screen.

Studies have found that the WURS has demonstrated reasonable psychometric properties. Internal consistency, four-week test retest reliability, and temporal stability were reported at .89, .81, and .68 for the WURS-61 and .88, .81, and .74 for the WURS-25, respectively (Rossini &

O' Connor, 1995). Wierzbicki (2005) reported similar reliability scores in a college population. The French and Italian forms have also demonstrated adequate reliability properties in the retrospective assessment of AD/HD in adults (Caci, Bouchez, & Bayle, 2010; Fossati et al., 2001).

Studies have failed to agree on a unified factor structure of the WURS. Thus, argument exists over the WURS' score validity for diagnosis. Stein et al. (1995) found that two different five-factor models for men and women best fit the data. The factors for men included conduct problems, learning problems, stress/intolerance, attention problems, and poor social skills/awkwardness, which accounted for 72% of the variance. The factors for women included dysphoria, impulsive/conduct problems, learning problems, attention and organization, and unpopular, which together accounted for 71% of the variance.

Recent studies have proposed a three-factor structure. McCann, Scheele, Ward, and Roy-Byrne (2000) found that dysthymia, oppositional/defiant behavior, and school problems accounted for 59.4% of the variance in adults referred for diagnostic screening. Internal consistency across these factors was reported at $\alpha = .95$. Adequate discriminant validity was obtained with only the school problems factor, which demonstrated reasonable specificity at 72%, yet poor sensitivity. In this study, the WURS positively screened half of those without AD/HD. McCann et al. failed to recommend the WURS for AD/HD diagnosis as the factors also measure depression and conduct problems, which may account for additional disorders.

Caci et al. (2010) found that impulsivity/temper, inattentiveness, and mood/self-esteem factors best fit the data for a sample of university students and parents referred for their child's diagnosis. Internal consistencies for the individual factors ranged from .85 to .92. Diagnostic accuracy was not reported and researchers recommended the WURS for adult diagnosis. Convergent validity with the ASRS was found to be moderate at .507. This relatively low correlation is expected as the ASRS measures symptoms in adulthood while the WURS is based on memory recall of childhood symptoms.

The WURS is best used as a supplementary instrument to aid in adult AD/HD diagnosis. The WURS has demonstrated exceptional reliability; however, the argument over the internal structure of the instrument poses a threat to the validity. The emerging factors appear to measure emotional and behavioral disturbances that may best account for other diagnoses rather than AD/HD in childhood. Therefore, researchers have cautioned that scores from this instrument may not be valid for diagnosis (McCann et al., 2000). In addition to weak validity evidence, a major disadvantage of this instrument is the use of retrospective assessment, as recollection may be characteristically faulty (Mackin & Horner, 2005). Clinicians should be aware of the shortcomings of the WURS and should strive to use instruments with sound psychometric properties.

Vanderbilt AD/HD Diagnostic Rating Scale—Parent and Teacher Version

The Vanderbilt AD/HD Diagnostic Rating Scale (VADRS) Parent (VADPRS) and Teacher Rating Scales (VADTRS) can be found online at http://www.brightfutures.org/mentalhealth/pdf/professionals/bridges/AD/HD.pdf and http://www.chironeuroindy.com/AD/HD-assessment-tools.htm, and are available for printing at http://www.childrens hospital.vanderbilt.org/interior.php?mid=5734. The VADRS has a parent and teacher form to assess AD/HD and related behaviors or symptoms in children. The items are presented at a third grade reading level.

The VADPRS contains 47 items, which assess the child's behaviors related to inattention, hyperactivity/impulsivity, oppositional defiant disorder (ODD), conduct disorder (CD), anxiety, and depression (Wolraich et al., 2003). The parent version also contains eight performance items. Four items assess the child's relationships in terms of peers, siblings, parents, and organized activities. The remaining four items ask the parents to rate the child's overall academic performance in math, reading, and written expression.

The VADTRS contains 35 items to measure behaviors related to inattention, hyperactivity/impulsivity, ODD, CD, anxiety, and depression (Wolraich, Feurer, Hannah, Baumgaerterl & Pinnock, 1998). The teacher version also contains eight performance items. Five items assess the child's classroom behaviors in terms of relationships with their peers, following directions, disrupting class, completion of assignments, and organization skills. The remaining three items ask the teacher to rate the child's overall academic performance in math, reading, and written expression.

Parents and teachers are to rate the severity of the child's behavior on a four-point scale ranging from 0–3: never (0), occasionally (1), often (2), and very often (3). Items rated with a two or three (often or very often) are considered clinically significant for diagnosis. For the performance section, parents and teachers are to rate the child's behavior on a five-point scale ranging from 1–5 (problematic to above average). A rating of one or two (problematic) for any item indicates the presence of a clinically significant impairment for diagnosis.

Clinically significant behaviors are totaled and compared to *DSM* criteria. For both the parent and teacher version, interpretations for inattentive, hyperactive, and combined presentation follow *DSM* criteria (http://www.brightfutures.org/mentalhealth/pdf/professionals/bridges/AD/HD.pdf). Children are diagnosed as predominately inattentive presentation if six or more behaviors and one performance item are clinically significant on items one to nine. Children are diagnosed as predominately hyperactive-impulsive presentation if six or more behaviors and one performance item are clinically significant on items 10–18. The combined subtype requires that these criteria be met for both inattentive and hyperactive-impulsive presentations.

Preliminary psychometric studies have reported satisfactory results. Internal consistency ranged from .94–.95 for the parent version and .90–.94 for the teacher version in a referred population of school-age children (Wolraich et al., 2003). A two-factor model of the parent version was found to be consistent with *DSM-IV* criteria as inattention and hyperactive/impulsive factors emerged. The teacher version contained a four-factor model. Concurrent validity with the Computerized Diagnostic Interview Schedule for Children (C-DISC-IV) was reported at $r = .79$.

The Vanderbilt is recommended for diagnosis in research studies. Further studies are needed to investigate the validity of the scales in the general and clinical population. Initial studies support the structured assessment as it is a time-efficient alternative to lengthy interview diagnostic practices.

SWANSON, NOLAN, AND PELHAM IV RATING SCALE (SNAP-IV)

The Swanson, Nolan, and Pelham rating scale (SNAP-IV) was designed to assess AD/HD, ODD, and other general pathological symptoms in school-age children (Bussing et al., 2008). The instrument has been used in several studies including the Multimodal Treatment Study of Children for AD/HD (MTA Cooperative Group, 1999a, 1999b). Several versions of the instrument with a varying number of items are available online. The 90-item instrument and scoring instructions can be accessed online at http://www.AD/HD.net/.

The long version contains 90 items and should take 30 minutes to complete. For AD/HD assessment, items include nine inattention and nine hyperactivity/impulsivity and a summary item for each (http://www.AD/HD.net/). For ODD assessment, items include eight *DSM-IV* related criteria, one *DSM-III-R* related criteria, and a summary item. The instrument includes 10 items from the Connor's Index Questionnaire and the Iowa Connor's Questionnaire to measure further childhood problems. An additional 40 items related to other possible childhood diagnoses are used as rule out criteria. Lastly, 10 items from the Swanson, Kotkin, Agler, Mylnn, and Pelham (SKAMP) rating scale ask the respondent to rate the severity of the child's classroom behaviors. Specific scoring instructions are provided on the website (http://www.AD/HD.net/). Scores for each item are summed and divided by the number of items in each subset, which is referred to as the average rating-per-item (ARI). Subscore ARIs are considered clinically significant at the 95th percentile.

The short version contains 26 items; 18 items pertain to AD/HD criteria with nine items related to inattention, nine items related to hyperactivity/impulsivity, and eight items related to ODD symptoms (Bussing et al., 2008). The form should take no longer than ten minutes to complete. Parents and teachers are asked to respond to symptom criteria on a four-point rating scale. Response ratings range from 0–3: (0) not at all; (1) just a little; (2) quite a bit; and (3) very much. The ARI is used for the six subscales for parent and teacher ratings of inattention, hyperactivity/impulsivity, and ODD (http://AD/HD.net/snap-iv-instructions.pdf).

A lack of published psychometric data is available to support the use of the 90-item SNAP-IV version. Initial psychometric reports support the reliability of the SNAP-IV short version. High internal reliability was reported for both parent and teacher ratings of the 26-item instrument, with alphas of .94 and .97, respectively (Bussing et al., 2008). Internal reliability reports for parent subscales were .90 for inattention, .79 for hyperactivity/impulsivity, and .89 for ODD. Internal reliability for teacher subscales was reported with alphas of .96, .92, and .96. Moderate inter-rater reliability between parents and teachers was reported at .49 for inattention, .43 for hyperactivity/impulsivity, and .47 for ODD, which is expected of AD/HD rating scales. A three-factor structure was confirmed for the three subscales.

While The SNAP-IV is available for free use and has been used in popular AD/HD treatment studies, psychometric data is lacking in the literature. Initial reliability data supports the use of the SNAP-IV short version for screening childhood AD/HD and ODD. Further psychometric studies and normative data are needed to support both the 26-item and the 90-item version available on the website for use in the general population.

Oregon Adolescent Depression Project—Conduct Disorder Screener

The Oregon Adolescent Depression Project–Conduct Disorder Screener (OADP-CDS) was developed as a screening instrument for Conduct Disorder. This brief self-report instrument was designed to assess the frequency of delinquent behaviors in older adolescents. This tool has been used in research studies, but has yet to gain popularity.

The OADP-CDS contains six-items: (1) I broke rules at home; (2) I broke rules at school; (3) I got into fights; (4) I skipped school; (5) I ran away from home; and (6) I got into trouble for lying or stealing (Lewinsohn, Rohde, & Farrington, 2000, p. 889). This screening test should take an individual less than five minutes to complete. Respondents are asked to rate the frequency of the occurrence on a four-point scale from 1–4: (1) rarely or none at this time; (2) some or little of the time; (3) occasionally or moderate amount of time; or (4) most or all the time. Items are summed for a single score that may range from six (no indication of frequent behaviors) to 24 (maximum indication of behaviors).

Initial psychometric evidence supports the OADP-CDS for research on conduct disorder. Significant gender differences were found with males reporting more frequent behaviors, which was expected because conduct disorder prevalence rates among males are higher in the general population (Lewinsohn et al., 2000). Acceptable internal consistency alphas for females were reported at .72 for females and .78 for males. Highly significant intra-class coefficients were found at .38 for females and .32 for males. The OADP-CDS was compared with the Center for Epidemiological Studies–Depression (CES-D) instrument to demonstrate discriminant validity and confirmed its utility as a specific Conduct Disorder screener rather than a general psychopathology assessment. Significant correlations were found with delinquent and aggressive scales on the Youth Self Report (YSR) and the Child Behavior Checklist (CBCL). The instrument was also found to accurately predict cases of antisocial personality disorder in 75% of the sample. Those with a prior diagnosis of oppositional defiant disorder (ODD) were also found to score higher on the OADP-CDS.

Optimal cut scores were determined using receiver operating characteristic (ROC) analysis. For the general population, a cut score of nine is recommended with .75 sensitivity, .72 specificity, .085 positive predictive value (PPV), and .98 negative predictive value (NPV) (Lewinsohn et al., 2000). A cut score of nine obtained a 73% classification rate. For males, an optimal cut score of 10 is suggested with .75 sensitivity, .76 specificity, .144 PPV, .983 NPV, and a 76% classification rate. For females, an ideal cut score of eight is suggested with .67 sensitivity, .64 specificity, .031 PPV, .991 NPV, and a 64% classification rate. Researchers found that the screening efficacy of the OADP-CDS was similar to the Youth Self Report (YSR) and the Child Behavior Check List (CBCL) (Achenbach & Rescorla, 2001).

The OADP-CDS demonstrates promising efficacy as a self-screening instrument, with older adolescents, for conduct disorder. Initial psychometric evidence confirms its utility as a screening instrument in research studies. While the instrument has been used primarily in research settings, the promised confidentiality of anonymous reporting could have protected against response bias. In clinical settings, the perceived judgment of socially unacceptable responses could influence client ratings. Lewinsohn et al. (2000) caution against the use of the OADP-CDS as a diagnostic tool, as it demonstrated low positive predictive value.

Children's Yale Brown Obsessive Compulsive Disorder Scale

The Children's Yale Brown Obsessive Compulsive Disorder Scale (CY-BOCS) is considered the gold standard in assessing symptom severity of children diagnosed with obsessive compulsive disorder (OCD) (Storch et al., 2004). The semi-structured assessment should be clinician administered to both the parent and child. A supplementary OCD behavior checklist is used prior to assessing severity to determine the nature of the past and current symptoms. The checklist and the assessment tool can be accessed, for free, online at http://www.stlocd.org/handouts/CY-BOC-1-6.pdf.

The CY-BOCS Symptom Checklist (CY-BOCS-SC) contains eight categories of obsessions and nine categories of compulsions (http://www.stlocd.org/handouts/CY-BOC-1-6.pdf). The clinician inquires about the symptoms with the parent and child and simply marks whether the behavior occurred in the past and/or if it is still occurring. The CY-BOCS contains 10 items which measure the severity of obsessions and compulsions within the last week. Five questions are asked about the experience of obsessions and the same five questions are replicated for inquiry of compulsions. The items relate to impact on normal functioning and are as follows: time spent engaging in, interruption due to, suffering related to, struggle against, and control over, obsessions and compulsions (Storch et al., 2004). The clinician asks both the parent and child to rate the severity of their experience of OCD symptoms on a five-point scale from 0–4: none (0); mild (1); moderate (2); severe (3); or extreme (4). Items are summed for total scores ranging from 0 to 40. Interpretations of scores are based on the following categories: 0–7, subclinical; 8–15, mild; 16–23, moderate; 24–31, severe; and 32–40, extreme.

Researchers have provided initial psychometric support for the use of the CY-BOCS-SC. Internal consistency coefficients varied according to symptom cluster from .50 to .81 (Gallant et al., 2008). The CY-BOCS-SC displayed good to excellent convergence with the Anxiety Disorders Interview Schedule parent version (ADIS-IV-P). The CY-BOCS-SC also demonstrated adequate discriminative validity with measures of depression, anxiety, and trichotillomania. Researchers supported the use of the CY-BOCS-SC to evaluate the manifestations of OCD in the client.

Psychometric reports of the CY-BOCS provide evidence of score reliability and validity. High internal consistency for obsessive and compulsive scales and total score were reported at .80, .82, and .90, respectively (Storch et al., 2004). Inter-scale correlations between obsessive and compulsive scales were reported at .81, between total score and obsessive scale at .95, and total score and compulsive scale at .95. Good test-retest reliability for approximately 41 days was reported with intra-class coefficients at .70 for obsessive scales, .76 for compulsive scales, and .79 for total scores. Significant differences were found between the first and second testing, with the second test scores lower, which is expected based on testing effects. High convergent validity was found with the clinician rated Tourette's Disorder Scale—Parent Rating of OCD (TODS-PR-OCD) at .70 and the Clinical Global Impression (CGI) scale at .75. Reasonable convergent validity was found with scales of depression, aggression, and AD/HD. Adequate divergent validity was found with measures of anxiety and tic disorders.

The CY-BOCS Child Report form (CY-BOCS-CR) and the CY-BOCS Parent Report form (CY-BOCS-PR) have also been developed and validated for complementary use with the CY-BOCS. The self-report items contain parallel language from the CY-BOCS with the addition of prompts where the clinician would have asked a question. Prior to the obsessive or compulsive symptoms section, the prompt asks parents and children to rate the severity based on their preoccupying thoughts or the habits that they can't stop repeating. High internal consistency for the CY-BOCS-CR and CY-BOCS-PR were reported at .87 and .86, respectively (Storch et al., 2006). Convergent validity with the CY-BOCS was reported at .72 with the parent version and .58 with the child version. Acceptable divergent validity was displayed with both parent and child rating scales. Researchers supported the use of the self-report scales to gather additional information, to use for treatment monitoring, or to use in the case that a clinician is unavailable.

The CY-BOCS-SC, CY-BOCS, CY-BOCS-CR, and the CY-BOCS-PR are all validated instruments to use in the assessment of OCD symptom presence and severity in children. The CY-BOCS-SC provides useful information for researchers and clinicians alike about the features of the disorder that the client has encountered. The short nature of the CY-BOCS renders the instrument useful for research and clinical practice.

The addition of child and parent self-report instruments is also essential, as it can cross-validate the clinician's ratings.

THE HOARDING RATING SCALE—INTERVIEW

The Hoarding Rating Scale–Interview (HRS-I) was designed to assess the presence and severity of compulsive hoarding. It should be clinician administered and takes 5–10 minutes to complete. It can be accessed, for free, online at http://www.ocfoundation.org/uploadedFiles/Hoarding/Resources/Hoarding%20Rating%20Scale%20with%20interpret.pdf.

The clinician asks the participant five questions which assess the features of compulsive hoarding (Tolin, Frost, & Steketee, 2010). The items inquire about the individual's trouble using living areas due to buildup of items, struggle to part with these items, extreme procurement of items, substantial distress due to hoarding actions, and disruptions in daily functioning as a result of hoarding behaviors. The participant is asked to rate the severity of their symptoms on a nine-point scale from 0–8, with (0) indicating no difficulty; (1–2) mild; (3–4) moderate; (5–6) severe; and (7–8) extreme difficulty. Items are summed for a total score which may range from 0 to 40. An optimum total cut-off score for indication of the presence of compulsive hoarding was found at 14 with specificity and sensitivity at 97%. Individual item optimal cut-off scores were also found at 3 for items one, four and five; 4 for item two; and 2 for item three.

Initial psychometric reports indicate significant score reliability and validity of the HRS-I. High internal consistency was reported at .97 and inter-item correlations ranged from .77 to .91 (Tolin et al., 2010). Test-retest reliability ranged from one to 12 weeks across administrations from the clinic to the home, yet still was reported high with a total of .96. The HRS-I was able to successfully discriminate between those with hoarding behaviors and those with OCD. Convergent validity was found with the Clutter Image Rating (CRI) scale at .72 in the clinic and .78 in the home; with the Saving Inventory–Revised (SI-R) at .91 in the clinic and .94 in the home; and with the Obsessive Compulsive Inventory–Revised (OCI-R) hoarding subscale at .89 in the clinic.

The HRS-I has been validated for the clinical assessment of the presence of hoarding behaviors. The addition of severity indication may also render the instrument useful for treatment monitoring; however, further research is needed to confirm this use. As hoarding has recently been acknowledged as a separate disorder, rather than a feature of OCD, this instrument is vital for clinicians and researchers for its practical usefulness, because it effectively discriminates hoarding from OCD.

Various Additional Online Measures

Many online resources are available for screening of impulse, disruptive, and obsessive compulsive disorders in addition to the aforementioned tools. However, there is no psychometric evidence to support the use of these surveys. These assessments are best used for personal inquiry or to prompt individuals to seek professional care.

- Oppositional Defiant Disorder Test (nine-item questionnaire for parent assessment of child behavior) http://www.organizedwisdom.com/Quiz/Oppositional_Defiant_Disorder_Test
- How to Tell if Your Child has Oppositional Defiant Disorder - ODD (symptom checklist for parents) http://www.squidoo.com/ODD
- Does Your Child Have Conduct Disorder? (parent questionnaire) http://addAD/HDadvances.com/CDtest.html
- Do you have Body Dysmorphic Disorder? (self-test) http://www.pamguide.com.au/anxiety/bdd_test.php
- Do you have Trichotillomania? (self-test) http://www.pamguide.com.au/anxiety/ttm_test.php

CHAPTER 6

Assessment of Disorders on the Autistic and Schizophrenic Spectrums

AUTISM SPECTRUM DISORDER

Recent trends showcasing increasing prevalence rates of autism spectrum disorders (ASD) have sparked a profusion of research designed to elucidate the reasons behind the sudden upsurge. ASDs have increased worldwide, and any international differences in prevalence rates are largely due to methodological differences in study designs (Zaroff & Uhm, 2012). At this point, it is unclear whether increased prevalence rates are due to a true increase or expanded diagnostic criteria and improved case-finding (Charman, 2011; Leonard et al., 2010). It is highly probable that increased public awareness and services have also played a role in the observed rise in prevalence rates (Saracino, Noseworthy, Steiman, Reisinger, & Fombonne, 2010). Given that increased prevalence rates are likely due to a combination of the aforementioned factors, the real concern is not *why* prevalence rates are rising but what can be done to appropriately meet this increasingly critical public health concern.

Currently, autism spectrum disorders are estimated to affect approximately 1 in 100 children (Baron-Cohen et al., 2011), although some place this estimate slightly higher, at 2.2 to 2.6 in 100 children (Kim et al., 2011; Saracino et al., 2010). Those significantly more likely to be diagnosed with ASD include Caucasians (Zaroff & Uhm, 2012), those of a higher socioeconomic status (Durkin et al., 2010), and boys (Baron-Cohen et al., 2011). Boys are four times more likely to be diagnosed with ASD than girls (Mitka, 2010). Some argue that boys are more likely to be diagnosed because autism is an extreme expression of the male brain, rendering boys biologically predisposed to be nearer the diagnostic threshold than girls (Baron-Cohen et al.). Others argue that, since assessment of ASD has been conducted with predominantly male samples, the current diagnostic criteria and assessments may not be appropriate for females, in whom ASD might present differently (Rivet & Matson, 2011).

Clinicians are becoming increasingly adept at helping those with ASD achieve monumental gains in social and emotional functioning. Numerous researchers have identified the exigency of early intervention in order for children to attain the best possible outcomes (Mitka, 2010; Wilkinson, 2010). Early intensive behavior intervention is effective for many children with ASD. Given that those with ASD often have comorbid diagnoses of anxiety disorders, mood disorders, and AD/HD (Rosenberg, Kaufmann, Law, & Law, 2011), it is critical that these children are identified as soon as possible, in order to ensure that they receive treatment for all of their potential diagnoses. Although some children are not identified as potentially meeting the criteria for ASD until they are of school age, diagnoses of ASD can be made as early as age two. These diagnoses made as early as age two years demonstrate acceptable levels of stability (Kleinman, Ventola et al., 2008), so early screening and diagnosis is recommended as a reliable method of ensuring children with ASD have early access to intervention and, hopefully, more favorable results.

Diagnostic criteria for ASD have undergone substantial revision in the *DSM-5* (APA, 2013). All of the sub-classifications, including autism disorder, Asperger's disorder, and pervasive developmental disorder—not otherwise specified, covered in the *DSM-IV-TR* have been removed in favor of subsuming all of these classifications under a single dimensional, diagnostic heading - autism spectrum disorder. Although many researchers recognize that this change effectively evinces the many shared features among the various sub-classifications (Charman, 2011), the unification of these many diverse disorders into one comprehensive diagnosis has raised some concerns, namely that, although the lumping together of sub-classifications into ASD will likely eliminate over-diagnosis at the milder end of the spectrum, overall prevalence rates may actually increase due to false positives engendered by the new view of unified disorders as an undifferentiated categorical spectrum (Barrett &

Fritz, 2010). An important advantage of the proposed changes is that previously unqualified children will likely be able to access the special education services they need. As scientists increase their understanding of the etiology of autism, new breakthroughs in optimal diagnostic criteria and categories are sure to follow.

According to the most recent revisions, ASD is characterized by the presence of both (a) persistent deficits in social communication and social interaction and (b) restrictive and repetitive patterns of behavior (APA, 2013). Insufficiencies in social communication and social interaction must manifest as deficits in all three of the following: (a) social-emotional reciprocity, (b) nonverbal communicative behaviors, and (c) the development and maintenance of relationships. Restricted, repetitive, patterns of behavior, interests, or activities must be manifested by at least two of the following: (a) stereotypy in speech, movements, or object use, (b) rigid adherence to behaviors or routines, (c) intense restricted interests, or (d) sensory hyperreactivity or hyporeactivity. A severity level of one, two, or three will be assessed for both social deficits and restrictive and repetitive patterns of behavior. Furthermore, these symptoms must present in early childhood and must together limit and impair daily functioning.

Schizophrenia and Other Delusional Disorders Encountered in Clinical Practice

The disorders classified in the "Schizophrenia and Other Delusional Disorders" category in the *DSM-5* are organized to reflect increasing severity of psychopathology (APA, 2013). Thus, schizotypal personality disorder, delusional disorder, and brief psychotic disorder compose the least severe end of the spectrum, while schizophrenia, psychotic disorder not otherwise classified, and catatonic disorder not otherwise specified represent the most severe psychopathology. Substance-induced psychotic disorder, psychotic disorder associated with another medical condition, catatonic disorder associated with another medical condition, schizophreniform disorder, and schizoaffective disorder comprise the middle of the schizophrenic spectrum, indicating moderate levels of severity. Each of these disorders features the presence of at least one psychotic symptom, such as hallucinations, delusions, disorganized thoughts/speech, catatonic/disorganized behavior, or a negative symptom like flattened affect or alogia.

Although the majority of these disorders are quite rare, the effects are so severely disabling that critical attention in this field is warranted. Schizotypal personality disorder (SPD) is the most common of the disorders in this category, with a 3.9 percent lifetime prevalence rate (Pulay et al., 2009). Males, black women, those with lower incomes, and those who have been separated, divorced, or widowed are more likely to be diagnosed with SPD. The risk of being diagnosed with SPD is significantly lower among Asian men. Diagnoses of SPD are often comorbid with diagnoses of bipolar I and II disorders, posttraumatic stress disorder, generalized anxiety disorder, borderline personality disorder, narcissistic personality disorder, and specific and social phobias.

Schizotypal personality disorder is characterized by both typical impairments in personality functioning and the presence of pathological personality traits (APA, 2013). For a diagnosis of schizotypal personality disorder to be warranted, impairments in personality functioning must include (a) impairments in self-functioning (confused/distorted identity or unrealistic/incoherent self-direction) and (b) impairments in interpersonal functioning (lack of empathy or impairments in developing intimate relationships). Five levels of self-interpersonal functioning impairment are delineated to differentiate varying levels of severity. Pathological personality traits must be identified in each of the following domains: (a) psychoticism, as characterized by eccentricity, cognitive and perceptual dysregulation, and unusual beliefs and experiences; (b) detachment, as characterized by restricted affectivity and withdrawal; and (c) negative affectivity, as characterized by suspiciousness. These impairments in personality functioning and trait expression must be stable and consistent across both time and situations, and cause cannot be attributed to developmental stage, socio-cultural environment, the physiological effects of a substance, or a general medical condition.

Although schizotypal personality disorder is the most common of all the disorders along this spectrum of psychopathy, schizophrenia undeniably receives the most attention in clinical and research ventures, likely due to its increased severity and debilitating chronicity. Approximately 5 out of every 1000 persons will be diagnosed with schizophrenia at some point in his or her lifetime (Goldner, 2003; Saha, Chant, Welham, & McGrath, 2005). Lifetime prevalence of schizophrenia is equal among males and females (Saha et al.). Higher prevalence rates have been observed among migrant groups and in developed nations, while prevalence rates are significantly lower among Asian populations (Goldner, 2003). Schizophrenia, in both its full and prodromal stages, is often comorbid with anxiety disorders, mood disorders, and substance/alcohol use disorders, especially cannabis use disorder (Bizzarri et al., 2009; Rosen, Miller, D'Andrea, McGlashan, & Woods, 2006).

Merely a generation ago, schizophrenia was blamed on poor parenting and dysfunctional families, but researchers now grasp the exceptional complexity of schizophrenia, advocating for understanding of schizophrenia as a brain disorder (Harrington, 2012). Although genetics likely play a prominent role in its development, attempts to identify specific anatomic correlates have been unsatisfactory (Dias, 2012). Dias recommended integrating glutamatergic hypotheses with white matter hypotheses in order to more accurately understand the etiology of schizophrenia from onset to chronification. Furthermore, Morgan et al. (2011) have proposed that risk factors in the environment may interact with genetic predispositions. These possible risk factors include prenatal complications, urbanicity, migration, ethnicity, stress, cannabis use, and family history of psychosis.

Given the abundance of evidence pointing to the physiological causes of this disorder, schizophrenia is often treated with both psychosocial and pharmacological treatment methodologies. Saha et al. (2005) estimated that current methods of treatment serve to reduce about 25 percent of the disease burden of schizophrenia. Recently, researchers found that atypical antipsychotic medications improve negative symptoms, affective symptoms, and cognitive functioning better than typical antipsychotics, but at the expense of dose-related increases in extrapyramidal symptoms (Lublin, Eberhard, & Levander, 2005). Furthermore, NMDA receptor modulators as adjuncts to antipsychotics have proved efficacious in treating the symptoms of schizophrenia (Singh & Singh, 2009). Cognitive-behavioral therapy (CBT) is efficacious in the treatment of schizophrenia as well, although therapeutic benefits are often not observed until a few months after termination of treatment (Sarin, Wallin, & Widerlööv, 2011). The more sessions of CBT a client receives, the better the likelihood of positive outcomes. Although CBT is commonly and effectively used for the treatment of schizophrenia, it must be acknowledged that some recent reviewers have questioned the true efficacy of CBT in its treatment (Morrison, 2009). Overall, treatment is most effective if it is begun in the initial stages of schizophrenia, but unfortunately more than half of those with schizophrenia do not receive appropriate care (World Health Organization, 2012).

Schizophrenia is characterized by the presence of at least two of the following, each of which must be present for a significant portion of a one-month period: (a) delusions, (b) hallucinations, (c) disorganized speech, (d) abnormal psychomotor behavior (e.g., catatonia), or (e) diminished expressions of affect (APA, 2013). At least one of the two criteria needed for Criterion A should include either delusions, hallucinations, or disorganized speech. Criterion B states that one or more major areas of functioning, such as school, work, interpersonal relations, or self-care, must have fallen markedly below the level of functioning achieved prior to onset of the disorder. Continuous signs of the disturbance must persist for a minimum of six months, and may include periods of prodromal or residual symptoms. Disturbance due to schizoaffective disorder, depressive or bipolar disorder with psychotic features, and the direct physiological effects of a substance or general medical condition must all be ruled out as well. Finally, if an individual has a history of childhood onset of autistic disorder, another pervasive developmental disorder, or another communication disorder, schizophrenia is only diagnosed in addition to this prior diagnosis if prominent delusions or hallucinations are also present for at least one month, or less if successfully treated. Overall severity of various dimensions will be assessed on a zero to four scale. The inclusion of sub-types of schizophrenia has been eliminated in the *DSM-5*.

A major debate in the literature today focuses on the efficacy, validity, and ethical aspects of early intervention in psychotic disorders (Simmons & Hetrick, 2012). The broader literature on psychosis risk generally does not support the use of the term "prodrome," preferring instead "ultra high risk" or "psychosis risk syndrome" to more appropriately imply increased risk rather than inevitability (Jorm, 2011). Some researchers argue strongly against the identification and labeling of those deemed at risk for psychosis, believing that early stigmatization and demoralization present unnecessarily large risks (Raven, Stuart, & Jureidini, 2012). Others advocating against the use of prodromal diagnosis added that clinicians should treat symptoms as they currently present, rather than guessing as to the covert disorder lurking beneath the surface (Rosenman & Anderson, 2011), although recommended treatments do not seem to be based on assumptions of a hidden disease pathway (Jorm). Other researchers have added that the transition from a prodromal to a psychotic state is ill-defined and lacks validation (Yung, Nelson, Thompson, & Wood, 2010). As the debate over whether labeling people as "high risk" is beneficial or harmful to early intervention continues, it seems that the use of "psychosis risk syndrome" is most appropriate as a research, rather than a clinical, diagnosis (Jorm, 2011). Researchers continue to expand their knowledge about the diagnosis "attenuated psychosis syndrome," (APA, 2013).

Commonalities between Schizophrenia and Autism Spectrum Disorder

Children with autism were originally diagnosed under the classification of "schizophrenia–childhood type" until the two disorders were made separate in the *DSM-III* (Dvir & Frazier, 2011). Although the links between the two diagnostic categories were subsequently ignored for several decades, researchers have recently begun revisiting the commonalities between disorders on the autistic and schizophrenic spectrums. The most notable shared clinical features include social withdrawal, communication impairments, and theory of mind deficits (Dvir & Frazier, 2011; King & Lord, 2010). Autism and schizophrenia are mainly distinguished by the presence of paranoid ideation in those with a diagnosis on the schizophrenia spectrum (King & Lord, 2010). However, some have suggested that when those with autism face an activity change or disruption in their routine, they can appear thought-disordered and paranoid (Dvir & Frazier, 2011).

King and Lord (2010) have proposed that autism and schizophrenia may share a common pathogenesis but may differ in either the time of onset, level of severity, or, due to effects on different brain areas, phenotypic expression. Although exactly how the two disorders are linked remains unclear, research supporting the clinical and biological commonalities among disorders on the autism and schizophrenia spectrums is abundant (Dvir & Frazier, 2011). For instance, many childhood-onset diagnoses of schizophrenia were preceded by or comorbid with ASD. Furthermore, numerous researchers have demonstrated common developmental delays in language and motor stereotypies, shared genetic factors, similar gray matter volumes, and parallel mirror neuron functional deficits (Dvir & Frazier, 2011; King & Lord). Interestingly, both drugs currently used for the pharmacological treatment of autism were originally developed for the treatment of schizophrenia (King & Lord).

So, although disorders on the autistic and schizophrenic spectrums are clinically distinct, they overlap in numerous ways. Further establishment of the connection between disorders on both of these spectrums will likely enhance early identification and treatment (King & Lord, 2010). Thus, this chapter focuses on identifying the best available instruments used in screening and assessment of disorders on both the autistic and schizophrenic spectrum. It is hoped that future researchers will be able to clarify the link between disorders on these two spectrums and eventually develop unified screening instruments that account for their shared clinical features, in order to efficiently and accurately screen for disorders on both spectrums.

Highlights of Free-Access Instruments Used to Identify and Monitor Outcomes

A wide array of instruments is available to measure the presence and severity of ASD. Although these instruments were designed to assess a specific sub-classification of an ASD before they were unified under one diagnostic continuum, given the similarities in past and present diagnostic criteria all are likely still appropriate for screening and assessing autism dimensionally. Future researchers should seek to confirm this assumption.

The majority of instruments used to measure the presence, severity, and outcomes of schizophrenia are not free access. Of the few that are, the best instrument for the assessment of schizophrenia is recommended here. A summary of a promising new instrument is also included. Thus, this section provides summaries of recommended commonly used free-access instruments of the assessment of both autistic spectrum and schizophrenic spectrum disorders.

Modified Checklist for Autism in Toddlers

The Modified Checklist for Autism in Toddlers (M-CHAT) is a parent-report instrument designed to screen for ASDs in children aged 16–30 months (Robins, Fein, Barton, & Green, 2001). Given that ASDs have recently been condensed into one overarching diagnosis, this instrument is ideally suited to match updated *DSM-5* criteria because it assesses ASDs as a single comprehensive spectrum, rather than many separate disorders. Using the original Checklist for Autism in Toddlers (CHAT), which included a behavioral observation, Robins et al. and colleagues eliminated the observation portion and extended the number of parent-report items to encompass a broader range of autism spectrum disorders and increase the brevity and efficiency of instrument administration. The M-CHAT is widely used and highly respected today, and has been translated and validated for use in Spain, China, Japan, and various Arabic countries (Canal-Bedia et al., 2011; Eldin et al., 2008; Gong et al., 2011; Inada, Koyama, Inokuchi, Kuroda, & Kamio, 2011).

Originally designed for use in a pediatrician's office (Robins et al., 2001), parents and clinicians can now access the M-CHAT for free at https://m-chat.org/index.php. However, although no requirements exist for administration, results should be interpreted with the guidance of a health care professional, making the M-CHAT a Level B test. Completion of the M-CHAT requires approximately five to ten minutes. The M-CHAT is composed of 23 yes/no questions about the child's typical behavior which are scored on a pass/fail basis. Seven items assessing social relatedness and communication have been deemed "critical questions." If the child either fails any three questions or at least two "critical questions," the child has screened positively at risk for an ASD, and referral for a follow-up interview is warranted. The follow-up interview expands upon items which the child failed in order to ensure the accuracy of the original response. Children whose scores still meet either of the referral criteria after administration of the follow-up interview are recommended to pursue further developmental evaluation with a specialist. Thus, the M-CHAT is appropriate for use in screening both the general population and children already identified as "at risk" for ASD.

Plenty of evidence exists to support both the reliability and the validity of scores on the M-CHAT. Internal consistency coefficients are invariably reported to be high, ranging from .80 to .85 for total items and .74 to .83 for critical items (Gong et al., 2011; Robins et al., 2001; Snow & Lecavalier, 2008). Various researchers obtained interrater reliability coefficients ranging from .79 to .93 and test-retest reliability coefficients ranging from .77 to .99 (Gong et al., 2011; Inada et al., 2011). The sensitivity and specificity of total and critical scores on the M-CHAT are both high, with most researchers reporting values in excess of .70, although a few have found specificities as low as .38 (Eldin et al., 2008; Gong et al, 2011; Kozlowski, Matson, Worley, Sipes, & Horovitz, 2012; Robins et al.; Snow & Lecavalier, 2008). Given the critical importance of identifying all true positives, high sensitivity is of greater importance than high specificity. Furthermore, both sensitivity and specificity are enhanced with the use of the follow-up interview (Kleinman, Robins et al., 2008).

Evidence for the validity of scores on the M-CHAT is copious. Content validity is supported by the fact that item development was based on literature reviews, adaptations, for use with older children, of previously-validated instruments, and expert clinical experience (Robins et al., 2001). Convergent validity is evidenced by findings that scores on the M-CHAT correlate significantly with scores on the Child Autism Rating Scale (r = .58) (Inada et al., 2011) as well as scores on the Social Communication Questionnaire (r = .77) (Snow & Lecavalier, 2008), both similar screening instruments for ASD. M-CHAT scores also predict the performance of 18-month-old infants on tasks designed to evaluate theory of mind, an important construct in ASDs (Wright & Poulin-Dubois, 2012). Various researchers have reported that children who were later diagnosed with ASD obtained significantly higher scores on the M-CHAT than children who were not later diagnosed with ASD, lending support to predictive criterion-related validity (Inada et al., 2011; Kozlowski et al., 2012; Robins et al., 2001; Snow & Lecavalier, 2008; Ventola et al., 2007). However, Kozlowski et al. noted that the M-CHAT is better able to discriminate between those in the general population with or without a potential ASD than between those children at risk for an ASD or who have atypical development without the presence of an ASD. Conversely, Ventola and colleagues demonstrated that items on the M-

CHAT relating to joint attention and social responsiveness discriminated effectively between children with ASD and those with another type of developmental delay or language disorder. Thus, additional research into the efficacy of the M-CHAT in discriminating between children with an ASD and children with another type of developmental delay is warranted.

Like most screening instruments, the M-CHAT has both advantages and disadvantages. The most prominent advantage lies in the ability of the M-CHAT to quickly and efficiently screen for all levels of severity of a potential ASD diagnosis. Because parents can complete the instrument in the pediatrician's waiting room or on their home computers, the interpreter saves valuable administration time. Furthermore, recent research indicates that an abbreviated version of the M-CHAT may be sufficient for screening a population that has already been identified as at risk (Kozlowski et al., 2012). Additionally, although the M-CHAT is currently only appropriate for use with toddlers aged 16 to 30 months (Pandey et al., 2008), recent research indicates that it may be appropriate for use with children as old as 48 months (Snow & Lecavalier, 2008; Yama, Freeman, Graves, Yuan, & Campbell, 2012). However, although some found the M-CHAT to be appropriate and valuable for use among children with Down's syndrome (DiGuiseppi et al., 2010), others have found that concurrent motor, cognitive, vision, or hearing impairments can result in falsely elevated M-CHAT scores (Luyster et al., 2011). Finally, as with any parent-report instrument, objectivity and accuracy of parent responses cannot be guaranteed. However, given that parents have the greatest exposure to their child's behavior across various contexts and situations, they seem best suited to answer questions pertaining to the typical behavior of their child.

The M-CHAT is a commonly used and highly recommended screening instrument for ASD in children aged 16 to 30 months. The new, dimensional view of ASD in the *DSM-5* is supported by the fact that subgroups on the M-CHAT are differentiated based on different symptom severity rather than different symptom profiles. Thus, the M-CHAT conceptually aligns with the new diagnostic criteria in the *DSM-5* quite well. So, backed by strong psychometrics and ample evidence of the reliability and validity of scores, researchers using the M-CHAT can be confident that they are using the gold standard of free-access instruments in this field. The follow-up interview is a crucial step in identifying false positives after population screening (Kleinman, Robins et al., 2008). Finally, health care professionals must remember that they can save valuable time in administration by encouraging parents to fill out the questionnaire on their own, but they must always interpret the results themselves.

AUTISM SPECTRUM SCREENING QUESTIONNAIRE

The Autism Spectrum Screening Questionnaire (ASSQ) is a first-stage population screening instrument originally designed to screen for the symptoms of Asperger's disorder or high-functioning autism in order to make necessary referrals for further diagnostic evaluation (Ehlers, Gillberg, & Wing, 1999). The inability of the ASSQ to distinguish among various ASDs, coupled with the continuous distribution of scores (Posserud, Lundervold, & Gillberg, 2006), renders the ASSQ consistent with the new, dimensional view of ASDs proposed in the *DSM-5*. An extended version of the ASSQ, the ASSQ-REV, was recently constructed to better capture the presentation of ASDs in girls (Kopp & Gillberg, 2011). The ASSQ has been translated for use in multiple languages and is appropriate for use with boys and girls aged six to 17 years with mild mental retardation or normal intelligence. The ASSQ can be accessed for free at http://www.springerlink.com/content/h26q7u2323251347/fulltext.pdf.

No prior training is necessary to administer, score, and interpret the ASSQ, making it a Level A other-report instrument (Ehlers et al., 1999). Written at an 8th grade reading level, it is designed to be completed by both parents and teachers in approximately ten minutes (Campbell, 2005). The ASSQ is a 27-item checklist, to which parents or teachers are asked to indicate their child's abnormality by choosing "yes," "somewhat," or "no" for each item. Items cover social interaction, communication problems, restricted and repetitive behavior, and motor clumsiness, and are scored on a zero to two-point scale, with higher points indicative of greater abnormality. Individual item scores are summed to provide a total score ranging from zero to 54. Although some have supported the originally designated cut-points of 19 for parents and 22 for teachers (Ehlers et al., 1999; Mattila et al., 2009), other researchers have identified optimal cut-points for both parents and teachers of 15

(Posserud et al., 2006) and 17 (Posserud, Lundervold, & Gillenberg, 2009), while others believe that summing parent and teacher scores and using a combined cut-point of 30 is the best method (Mattila et al., 2009). A cut-point of 19 has been recommended for the 45-item ASSQ-REV (Kopp & Gillberg, 2011). Incontrovertibly, continued research is needed in order to confirm optimal cut-points for both parents and teachers. Currently, it seems that any score in excess of 15 is likely to indicate sub-threshold symptoms or potential ASD diagnosis, and thus further assessment is warranted.

Sufficient evidence for the reliability and validity of scores on the ASSQ has been presented. Internal consistency coefficients for the ASSQ were reported to be .89 for teachers and .86 for parents (Posserud et al., 2008). Internal consistency coefficients for the ASSQ-REV were also reported to be high across various population groups, with the majority in excess of .80 (Kopp & Gillberg, 2011). Test-retest reliability coefficients have been reported to range from .90 to .96 among both teachers and parents (Ehlers & Gillberg, 1993; Ehlers et al., 1999). Interrater reliability coefficients between parent and teacher reports have mostly been low to moderate, ranging from .26 to .79 (Ehlers et al., 1999; Ehlers & Gillberg; Mattila et al., 2009; Posserud et al., 2006). This discrepancy among ratings is not necessarily problematic, and is likely due to the importance of situational context in assessing subtle symptom presentation. The moderate to high sensitivity is generally superior to the low to moderate specificity of scores on the ASSQ (Ehlers et al., 1999; Mattila et al; Posserud et al., 2009) The best balance of sensitivity (1.0) and specificity (.92) was obtained at a cut-point of 15 for teachers and 18 for parents (Posserud et al., 2009).

Numerous researchers have demonstrated the convergent validity of the ASSQ via correlations with instruments designed to measure similar constructs. Scores on the ASSQ were significantly correlated with scores on the Rutter scale ($r = .75$ for parents, $r = .77$ for teachers) and scores on the Conners scale ($r = .58$ for parents, $r = .70$ for teachers), two scales designed to measure general behavioral problems in childhood (Ehlers et al., 1999). Total scores on the ASSQ and ASSQ-REV were highly correlated ($r = .98$), reinforcing the sound psychometric integrity of both instruments (Kopp & Gillberg, 2011). Posserud et al. (2008) confirmed a three factor structure of the ASSQ, comprised of social difficulties, motor/tics/OCD, and autistic style, for both parents and teachers. Moderate to high correlations were found among each of the factors and the peer problems factor on the Strengths and Difficulties Questionnaire, a broadband child psychiatric behavioral assessment.

The concurrent and predictive criterion-related validity of the ASSQ was supported by multiple researchers who found that higher scores on the ASSQ and ASSQ-REV were associated with clinical diagnoses of ASDs and that mean scores differed significantly among diagnostic groups of children with ASD, ADHD, and LD, and those without any type of psychiatric diagnosis (Ehlers et al., 1999; Kopp & Gillenberg, 2011).

The sole disadvantage of the ASSQ is the need for further research to confirm appropriate cut-points and the validity of scores. However, use of the ASSQ is advantageous for many reasons. First, the ASSQ is designed for use with both parents and teachers. Gathering information from both families and schools is essential for comprehensive screening, since autistic symptoms, especially subtle ones, are likely to vary across contexts, and may be more noticeable in school settings due to peer comparisons (Posserud et al., 2006; Posserud et al., 2009). Secondly, the ASSQ has been validated for use in community, clinical, and ASD-specific clinical settings (Campbell, 2005), and has been shown to accurately differentiate children with ASDs from those with AD/HD, behavior disorders, and learning disorders (Norris & Lecavalier, 2010). Although the ASSQ is unable to differentiate between Asperger's disorder and high-functioning autism (Mattila et al., 2009), this problem is inconsequential given the condensation of all autism spectrum disorders into one disorder of varying severity levels in the *DSM-5*. The ASSQ is able to identify both high and low functioning children, and it has performed similarly among boys and girls (Ehlers et al., 1999; Kopp & Gillberg, 2011; Mattila et al., 2009; Posserud et al., 2009), with a single exception in which boys scored significantly higher (Posserud et al., 2006).

Multiple researchers have sought continual improvement of the already superb ASSQ. Based on the results of factor analysis, Posserud et al. (2008) proposed that combining a flat cut-off score with an examination of the response profile could improve screening results. This suggestion, based on the fact that requiring a minimum score on the "autistic style" factor could weed out false identification of children with social difficulties due to other disorders, seems quite valuable, and necessitates further research for support. Additionally, the recent development of an extended version, the ASSQ-REV, designed to better capture the autism phenotype in girls, marks an important recognition of the fact that response profiles may differ significantly between boys and girls. By adapting an existing psychometrically-sound instrument to better screen for ASDs in girls, the developers of the ASSQ-REV have taken an important step forward in recognizing that screening for ASDs in girls may need to be different in order to accurately identify the rarer cases of ASDs in the female population.

The ASSQ has been hailed by many as showing promise, but in need of further examination (Campbell, 2005; Norris & Lecavalier, 2010), and it has been recommended as superior to, or on par with, other published and free-access common caregiver-completed scales for ASD screening in children over the age of three years. Given the continuous distribution of scores on the ASSQ, this screening instrument seems well-suited to identifying even the most subtly-pronounced cases of possible ASD. Thus, the ASSQ is recommended for use as a general population screen for the identification of potential symptoms of ASD in children and adolescents, and further inquiry into the validity of scores on the ASSQ is encouraged.

AUTISM SPECTRUM QUOTIENT

The Autism Spectrum Quotient (AQ) is one of the few instruments available for the assessment of the extent of autistic traits in adults with normal intelligence (Baron-Cohen et al., 2001). The AQ has been translated and validated in Japanese (Wakabayashi, Tojo, Baron-Cohen, & Wheelwright, 2004), German (Freitag et al., 2007), Dutch (Hoekstra, Bartels, Cath, & Boomsma, 2008), French-Canadian (Lepage, Lortie, Taschereau-Dumouchel, & Theoret, 2009), Turkish (Köse, Bora, Erermiş, & Aydin, 2010) and Italian (Ruta et al., 2012). The self-report AQ has also been adapted into parent-report versions for use with adolescents aged 10 to 15 years (AQ-Adol; Baron-Cohen, Hoekstra, Knickmeyer, & Wheelwright, 2006) and children aged 4 to 11 years (AQ-Child; Auyeung, Baron-Cohen, Wheelwright, & Allison, 2008). Numerous researchers have also developed abbreviated versions of the AQ (Allison, Auyeung, & Baron-Cohen, 2012; Hoekstra et al., 2011; Kurita, Koyama, & Osada,

2005). The AQ is appropriate for use with male and female adults over the age of 15 years. Children and adolescents under the age of 15 years should use the version corresponding to their age group. The AQ is available for free at http://aq.server8.org/; abbreviated and adapted versions can be found in the literature.

Advanced training for the administration, scoring, and interpretation of the AQ is not required. The AQ is composed of 50 items to which the respondent indicates degree of agreement on a four-point Likert scale, ranging from "definitely agree" to "definitely disagree" (Baron-Cohen et al., 2001). Ten questions each assess the domains of social skill, attention switching, attention to detail, communication, and imagination. Respondents receive one point for each endorsement, whether mild or strong, of an abnormal behavior; abnormality is defined as poor scores on all domains except attention to detail. Thus, scores can range from zero to 50. Specific items scoring zero or one point for certain responses are detailed in the original article. Scores are normally distributed among the general population (Hurst, Mitchell, Kimbrell, Kwapil, & Nelson-Gray, 2007), so higher scores are viewed as indicative of possession of a greater degree of characteristics associated with the autism spectrum. This conceptualization supports the dimensional view of ASD promoted in the *DSM-5*. More specifically, Baron-Cohen et al. (2001) suggest that scores of 32 or higher merit additional diagnostic evaluation for individuals experiencing distress as a result of their autistic traits.

Abundant support exists for the reliability and validity of scores on the AQ and its translated, adapted, and abbreviated versions. The majority of researchers have obtained both high overall internal consistency coefficients, ranging from .67 to .86, and moderate to high subscale internal consistency coefficients, ranging from .58 to .90 (Allison et al., 2012; Austin, 2004; Baron-Cohen et al., 2001; Hoekstra et al., 2008; Hoekstra et al., 2011; Hurst et al., 2007). Overall and subscale internal consistency coefficients for the child and adolescent versions of the AQ have been comparable or superior to those obtained for the original AQ (Auyeung et al., 2008; Baron-Cohen et al., 2006). Test-retest reliabilities ranged from .70 to .92 in general and clinical populations across all age-groups (Auyeung et al.; Baron-Cohen et al., 2001; Baron-Cohen et al., 2006; Hoekstra et al., 2008; Kose et al., 2010; Wakabayashi et al., 2004), with slightly lower estimates in abbreviated versions (Kurita et al., 2005).

Using the proposed cut-point of 32, researchers reported sensitivities and specificities in the mid to high .70s (Woodbury-Smith, Robinson, Wheelwright, & Baron-Cohen, 2005). Comparable or superior estimates have been reported for abbreviated versions (Kurita et al., 2005) and the children's version of the AQ (Auyeung et al., 2008). Notably, the latest 10-item versions of the child, adolescent, and adult AQ all achieved sensitivity and specificity values in excess of .88 with a cut-point of six, lending support to the use of abbreviated versions for efficient and accurate screening. Adults, children, and adolescents with ASD diagnoses have consistently scored significantly higher than control group individuals, providing evidence of concurrent validity (Allison et al., 2012; Auyeung et al, 2008; Baron-Cohen et al., 2001; Baron-Cohen et al., 2006; Hoekstra et al., 2008; Kurita et al., 2005; Wakabayashi, Baron-Cohen, Wheelwright, & Tojo, 2006; Wakabayashi et al., 2004; Wakabayashi et al., 2007; Woodbury-Smith et al., 2005). Although males in control groups have scored slightly, but not significantly, higher on the AQ than their female counterparts, no gender differences have been observed in those diagnosed with ASD (Austin, 2004; Auyeung et al., 2008; Baron Cohen et al., 2001; Baron-Cohen et al., 2006; Wakabayashi et al., 2006). However, Brugha et al. (2012) recently found that AQ scores were a weak predictor of diagnosed ASDs in a general population screening. AQ scores did not discriminate between various disorders on the autism spectrum, including Asperger's disorder, high-functioning autism, autistic disorder, and pervasive developmental disorder—not otherwise specified (PPD-NOS), but this is not problematic given the new dimensional conceptualization of ASDs in the *DSM-5* (Auyeung et al., 2008; Kurita et al., 2005).

Evidence in support of the factor structure of the AQ has been inconsistent. Although Baron-Cohen et al. (2001) created the AQ with a five-factor structure, subsequent researchers have found support for two (Hoekstra et al., 2008; Hoekstra et al., 2011), three (Austin, 2004; Hurst et al., 2007; Kose et al., 2010), and four factors (Auyeung et al., 2008; Stewart & Austin, 2009), as well as the original five-factor structure (Kloosterman, Keefer, Kelley, Summerfeldt, & Parker, 2011). However, most researchers agree on a social interaction and a patterns/attention to detail factor (Stewart & Austin, 2009), and many have found their new factors to be highly correlated with the original subscales of the AQ (Austin, 2004;

Auyeung et al., 2008). Hurst et al. suggested that deleting items that are unrelated to symptom domains could enhance the factor structure and brevity of the AQ. Future researchers should determine how best to condense items on the AQ in order to obtain a consistent factor structure.

The advantages of the AQ are manifold. The various translations and adaptations of the AQ have rendered it appropriate for use with male and female children, adolescents, and adults of various cultures. The similarity of AQ results across cultures showcases the widespread applicability of the AQ among diverse populations (Wakabayashi et al., 2006; Wakabayashi et al., 2007). Although many instruments in this field are unable to capture the expression of ASDs among females, the AQ is able to accurately identify females with ASD diagnoses (Baron-Cohen et al., 2001). Furthermore, the AQ has been used effectively with both general and at-risk populations, and can discriminate among those without a psychiatric diagnosis, those with schizophrenia, and those with autism (Wouters & Spek, 2011). Additionally, the robust psychometric properties reported for abbreviated versions of the AQ and their high correlations with the original AQ suggest that the use of shortened versions can enhance efficiency without compromising psychometric strength (Allison et al., 2012; Kurita et al., 2005).

The only problem with the AQ is the lack of support for a consistent factor structure. Future researchers should strive to enhance the validity of scores on the AQ by establishing a consistent factor structure in full or abbreviated versions. The finding that parents scored the AQ marginally higher than their child suggests that those with ASD may be prone to under-reporting their symptoms, but items on the AQ are specifically designed to identify even those who do not view their behavior as abnormal (Baron-Cohen et al., 2001). Thus, the AQ seems to be an accurate method of measuring the degree of ASD characteristics present among both those who self-report and those whose parents report for them.

The AQ is thus recommended as an efficient tool for both screening and conceptualizing where an individual falls on the autism spectrum. Consequently, the AQ has widespread potential applications in research, screening, and treatment planning. However, although many promote the AQ as a predictive instrument, Kurita et al. (2005) have suggested that the real utility of the AQ lies in its ability to rule out ASDs. The AQ should be used to gain knowledge about the expression of an ASD among children, adolescents, and adults.

PRODROMAL QUESTIONNAIRE—BRIEF VERSION

The Prodromal Questionnaire (PQ) was originally developed as a 92-item screen for prodromal and psychotic symptoms (Loewy, Bearden, Johnson, Raine, & Cannon, 2005), but was condensed into a 21-item Brief Version (PQ-B) to enhance efficiency and improve upon its psychometric properties (Loewy, Pearson, Vinogradov, Bearden, & Cannon, 2011). The PQ-B is a self-report questionnaire intended to identify adolescents and adults at risk for psychosis, and should be followed by a diagnostic interview to pinpoint the level of risk for a psychotic disorder. The PQ-B is currently appropriate mainly for use in a general mental health help-seeking population, and can be accessed in the literature (Loewy et al., 2011).

The PQ-B is designed for self-administration, but results should be interpreted by a trained clinician. Completion of the PQ-B requires approximately 10 minutes. Although the original PQ was comprised of four subscales, including positive symptoms, negative symptoms, disorganized symptoms, and general/affective symptoms, only items targeting positive symptoms were retained on the PQ-B due to their superior predictive ability (Loewy et al., 2011). Thus, the PQ-B is comprised of 21 dichotomously scored items which assess the experiences of respondents in the past month. For each item that the respondent endorses, he is asked to indicate the level of distress due to this experience via a follow-up five-point Likert-type item (1= strongly disagree; 2 = disagree; 3 = neutral; 4 = agree; 5 = strongly agree). Both total scores and distress scores are calculated upon completion of the questionnaire. To calculate the Total score, which can range from zero to 21, respondents receive one point for each "yes" response. To calculate the Distress score, each "yes" response is weighted by the level of distress and then all items are summed, resulting in a possible range of zero to 105 points. Various cut-points have been proposed to maximize sensitivity and specificity in diverse populations. Loewy and colleagues originally suggested that a Total score of three or greater, or a Distress score of six or greater, maximized these properties and warranted a follow-up diagnostic interview.

Adequate evidence in support of the reliability and validity of PQ-B scores exists, but, given its newness, additional research is certainly merited. Thus far, Loewy et al. (2011) have obtained an interrater reliability coefficient of .94 and an internal consistency coefficient of .85 for Total scores. Researchers using the PQ-B have been vexed by high sensitivities (.88 - .90) but low specificities (.44 - .68), leading some to suggest that while the PQ-B is effective for identifying those at high risk for developing psychosis, it is plagued by false identification of those with other mental health issues (Jarrett et al., 2012; Loewy et al., 2011). Thus, the PQ-B is currently most appropriate for use in a help-seeking population, rather than as a general population screen. However, the newest version of the PQ-B, the PQ-16, has demonstrated promising results with both sensitivity and specificity estimates of .87 when using a six-item cut-point (Ising et al., 2012). Furthermore, scores on the PQ-B have been shown to accurately predict diagnoses of prodromal and psychotic syndromes on the Structured Interview for Prodromal Syndromes (SIPS), and both Total and Distress scores differed significantly across diagnostic groups, providing support for the concurrent validity of scores on the PQ-B (Loewy et al., 2011). Convergent validity is evidenced by the moderate correlations obtained among Total and Distress scores and SIPS subscale scores, ranging from .50 to .65.

Although research on the psychometric properties of the PQ-B is still in its infancy, results thus far seem promising. Very few free-access instruments for the screening of those at risk for psychosis exist, yet early intervention is crucial for helping this population to obtain positive outcomes (Fiori Nastro et al., 2010; Yung, 2012). Thus, the PQ-B fills an important gap in helping mental health care providers to identify those in need of additional clinical interviews to evaluate psychosis risk (Ising et al., 2012; Loewy, Therman, Manninen, Huttunen, & Cannon, 2012). Furthermore, the PQ-B has proved useful in college student, prison, and mental health populations (Jarrett et al., 2012; Loewy, Johnson & Cannon, 2007; Loewy et al., 2011). Future researchers should serve to further extend the use of the PQ-B in additional populations, as its use is likely appropriate in a variety of help-seeking or at-risk populations. The PQ-B is additionally advantageous due to its self-report format - rather than an interview format - which is rare in the screening and assessment of psychotic disorders. Thus, administrators of the PQ-B can screen for those at risk for psychotic disorders without extensive demands on their time and clinical training background. Although the PQ-B is not as sensitive to differentiating between prodromal and fully developed psychosis, it is fully adept at distinguishing those without a diagnosis from those with either a prodromal or psychotic diagnosis (Loewy et al., 2011). Thus, the PQ-B is efficacious as a first-level screening instrument to identify those in need of further clinical assessment. However, it should be used with caution with adolescents since current at-risk criteria for the prediction of psychosis have been taken from research with adults and may not necessary apply to adolescents (Koch, Schultze-Lutter, Schimmelmann, & Resch, 2010).

Although additional research regarding the psychometric properties of the PQ-B is warranted, it is currently recommended as an innovative screening instrument for the early identification of distressing psychotic symptoms. The PQ-B should ideally be used to efficiently and effectively screen for psychotic disorders in help-seeking populations. However, although early identification of those at risk for psychosis is advantageous for helping them to attain earlier treatment and better outcomes, early symptoms have often proved difficult to use in predicting future psychosis (Fiori Nastro et al., 2010). Thus, researchers should be exceedingly cautious about unnecessary labeling and stigmatizing those deemed at risk for psychosis, and should focus mainly on the present symptoms rather than any perceived underlying illness trajectory.

Psychotic Symptom Rating Scales

The Psychotic Symptom Rating Scales were developed to assess the severity of various dimensions of auditory hallucinations and delusions (PSYRATS; Haddock, McCarron, Tarrier, & Faragher, 1999), and have since been translated into Spanish (Gonzalez, Sanjuán, Canete, Echánove, & Leal, 2003), Korean (Jung et al., 2007), and German (Kronmuller et al., 2011). Broken into two subscales, the auditory hallucinations scale and the delusions scale, the information gleaned from the PSYRATS is useful for treatment planning and outcome measurement, as well as for furthering researchers' understanding of the various dimensions of psychosis. Overall, the PSYRATS is an observer-rated semi-structured interview designed for use with male and female adults with diagnoses of schizophrenia or schizoaffective disorder. Now regarded as the gold standard in the assessment of psychotic symptoms, the PSYRATS can be accessed for free in the literature.

The PSYRATS is a Level C test, meaning it must be administered and interpreted either by an individual with a doctoral degree in psychology or a related discipline, or under the direct supervision of a qualified professional (Haddock et al., 1999). The auditory hallucinations (AH) subscale is composed of 11 items which assess frequency, duration, severity, distress, and specific symptom dimensions, while the delusions (D) subscale is composed of six items which assess dimensions of delusions. Items on both subscales are rated on a five-point Likert-type scale, ranging from zero to four. Clinicians are encouraged to consider the importance of both subscale totals and individual items when interpreting PSYRATS scores. This detailed, individualized approach to score analysis enables clinicians to pinpoint the focal areas and degrees of change among various symptom dimensions in order to judge the efficacy of previous treatments and specific dimensions to target for further improvement. Steel et al. (2007) have also supplied the distribution of scores on symptom severity to serve as reference data for clinicians seeking to supplement their clinical judgment with normative information.

Support for the reliability and validity of scores on the PSYRATS is abundant. Numerous researchers have obtained high internal consistency coefficients, ranging from .70 to .94 on each of the subscales (Hatton et al., 2005; Kronmuller et al., 2011). Scores on the PSYRATS also demonstrate excellent interrater reliability (Drake, Haddock, Tarrier, Bentall, & Lewis, 2007; Haddock et al., 1999; Kronmuller et al., 2011) and high test-retest reliability (r = .70 and rho = .99) (Drake, et al., 2007; Haddock et al., 1999; Hatton et al., 2005; Kronmuller et al., 2011).

Convergent validity was established by the numerous correlations found between scores on the PSYRATS and scores on similar measures of psychotic dimensions. The negative impact (NI) and negative dimensions (ND) subscales of the Subjective Experiences of Psychosis Scale (SEPS), a self-report instrument, correlated significantly with both the PSYRATS hallucinations subscale [r = .59 (NI) and r = .55 (ND)] and delusions subscale [r = .37 (NI) and r = .47 (ND)] (Haddock et al., 2011).

In support of convergent validity, scores on the hallucinations subscale of the PSYRATS have also correlated significantly with scores on the PANSS hallucination item (r = .47 - .81), the PANSS positive scale (r = .45), and the SAPS auditory hallucinations item (r = .27), while scores on the delusions subscale of the PSYRATS have correlated significantly with scores on the PANSS delusions item (r = .40 - .43), the PANSS Positive scale (r = .61), and the SAPS global rating of delusions (r = .35) (Drake et al., 2007; Hatton et al., 2005; Steel et al., 2007). Low to moderate correlations have also been obtained between the PSYRATS delusion scale and scores on the MMDAS and DDE, semi-structured interviews for the assessment of delusions, and the BABS, an assessment of delusional characteristics (Kronmuller et al., 2011). Correlations between PSYRATS scores and Hamilton Program for Schizophrenia Voices Questionnaire, a self-report measure of psychotic symptoms, at baseline, one week, eleven weeks, and six months later, all exceeded .73 (Kim et al., 2010).

As evidence of concurrent validity, PSYRATS AH scores have been shown to correlate highly with scores on diagnostic interviews for psychiatric diagnoses, including the PAS-ADD psychotic scores (r = .83) (Hatton et al., 2005). Additionally, groups diagnosed with psychosis have scored significantly higher on the PSYRATS AH subscale than other mental health problem groups.

The factor structure of the PSYRATS among various psychiatric populations appears to be quite stable (Kronmuller et al., 2011). The original three-factor structure of the AH subscale and two-factor structure of the D subscale (Haddock et al., 1999) were supported by recent researchers (Drake et al., 2007). Subsequent researchers have replicated the two-factor structure of the D subscale, but have found four factors to demonstrate a better fit on the AH subscale (Kronmuller et al. 2011; Steel et al., 2007). Although results thus far appear promising, additional research to support the factor structure of the PSYRATS is warranted.

Limited only by extensive, but necessary, training requirements for administration and interpretation, the advantages of the PSYRATS are manifold. Although mainly applicable to work with first episode and chronic schizophrenics (Drake et al., 2007; Haddock et al., 1999), the PSYRATS has been deemed suitable for use with diverse cultural populations (Steel et al., 2007), including adults with mild to moderate intellectual disabilities (Hatton et al., 2005). The amount of detail about psychotic dimensions supplied by responses on the PSYRATS enables clinicians to better understand these symptoms and thus adapt treatment accordingly (Drake et al., 2007). Therefore, PSYRATS can be used throughout treatment as a formative assessment of progress in order to ensure that clients are receiving the most efficacious treatment methodologies. Furthermore, the ability of the PSYRATS to measure distress, which is often overlooked in diagnostic measures, enables the clinician to assess treatment outcome based on change in distress (Steel et al., 2007). Given that the negative tone of auditory hallucinations are likely to predict the presence of psychosis, the attention paid to the content of hallucinations in the PSYRATS is undoubtedly a crucial diagnostic step (Daalman et al., 2011). Another notable advantage of the PSYRATS is the applicability of the delusions subscale to those with affective disorders (Kronmuller et al., 2011).

In summary, the PSYRATS is incredibly useful for measuring psychotic symptom dimensions in both research and clinical settings. Heralded as the "gold standard" in the assessment of psychotic symptoms, scores on the PSYRATS subscales and key relevant items can provide substantial insights into treatment planning and outcome assessment. Clinicians should consider breaking the identified factors on each of the two major subscales into small subscales for enhanced interpretation (Kronmuller et al., 2011). Overall, the substantial evidence of the reliability and validity of scores on the PSYRATS render it an intelligent choice for interviewer-rated assessment of psychotic symptom dimensions.

CHAPTER 7

Assessment of Eating Disorders

PRIMARY EATING DISORDERS COMMONLY ENCOUNTERED IN CLINICAL PRACTICE

Eating disorders are a pressing problem and have become increasingly present and diversified. The four main types of eating disorders recognized by the most recent edition of the *Diagnostic and Statistical Manual of Mental Disorders* (*DSM-5*; APA, 2013) include anorexia nervosa, bulimia nervosa, binge eating disorder, and eating disorder not otherwise specified. Other feeding and eating disorders included in the *DSM-5* include pica, rumination disorder, and avoidant/restrictive food intake disorder, which are less common.

Anorexia nervosa is characterized by: (a) restricted energy intake resulting in significantly low body weight; (b) fear of gaining weight; and (c) body weight or shape disturbance, or unwillingness to acknowledge the seriousness of the condition (APA, 2013). Those who meet all three of these criteria are then classified as Binge Eating/Purging Type or Restricting Type, depending on whether or not they have engaged in recurrent episodes of binge eating or purging behavior, respectively, during the last three months. Amenorrhea, the absence of menstrual periods, has been a long-standing diagnostic criterion for anorexia nervosa, but has been removed in the *DSM-5* due to evidence indicating that many individuals meet all other criteria but report some menstrual activity.

Bulimia nervosa is characterized by: (a) recurrent episodes of binge eating; (b) recurrent compensations to prevent weight gain; (c) both a and b occur at least once a week for three months; (d) poor body image; and (e) not limited to occurrence during episodes of anorexia nervosa (APA, 2013). Binge eating, the first criterion, is defined as eating an amount of food that is definitely larger than most people would eat during a similar time period and under similar circumstances, and it is characterized by a sense of lack of control over eating during the episode. The purging and non-purging subtypes of the *DSM-IV* (APA, 1994) have been eliminated.

Binge eating disorder is characterized by: (a) recurrent episodes of binge eating; (b) association with three or more of the following: eating much more rapidly than normal; eating until feeling uncomfortably full, eating large amounts of food when not feeling physically hungry, eating alone because of feeling embarrassed by how much one is eating, or feeling disgusted with oneself, depressed, or very guilty afterwards; (c) marked distress regarding binge eating; (d) occurrence of binge eating at least once a week, on average, for three months; and (e) the binge eating is not associated with the recurrent use of inappropriate compensatory behavior and does not occur exclusively during the course of anorexia nervosa, bulimia nervosa, or avoidant/restrictive food intake disorder (APA, 2013).

Feeding and eating conditions not elsewhere classified, previously known as eating disorder not otherwise specified (EDNOS), provides brief descriptions of several conditions of potential clinical significance that do not meet criteria for feeding and eating disorders (APA, 2013). These various conditions include atypical anorexia nervosa, sub-threshold bulimia nervosa, sub-threshold binge eating disorder, purging disorder, night eating syndrome, and other feeding or eating condition not elsewhere classified.

Although most eating disorders appear to be relatively rare, commonly used interview methods may underestimate the prevalence of eating disorders due to minimization and denial of symptoms (Hudson, Hiripi, Pope, & Kessler, 2007). Eating disorders affect individuals of various cultures and ethnicities (Hoek & van Hoeken, 2003), although diagnosis of anorexia nervosa occurs most often in industrialized countries (Reijonen, Pratt, Patel, & Greydanus, 2003). Women are 10 times more likely to be diagnosed with an eating disorder than men (Hoek & van Hoeken, 2003; Reijonen, Pratt, Patel, & Greydanus, 2003).

Hudson et al. (2007) estimate the lifetime prevalence of anorexia nervosa (AN) to be 0.9% among women and 0.3% among men. This is similar to other estimates (Reijonen et al., 2003), although some researchers have reported prevalence rates closer to 2% (Keski-Rahkonen et al., 2007; Wade, Bergin, Tiggemann, Bulik, & Fairburn, 2006). Prevalence rates of anorexia nervosa are reported to be 0.3% among adolescents (Hoek & van Hoeken, 2003; Swanson, Crow, le Grange, Swendsen, & Merikangas, 2011).

Bulimia nervosa (BN) is estimated to be more common than anorexia nervosa. Hudson et al. (2007) estimate the lifetime prevalence of bulimia nervosa to be 1.5% among women and 0.5% among men. Previous researchers have obtained similar lifetime prevalence estimates internationally, ranging from 1.0% to 3.0% for women (Hoek & van Hoeken, 2003; Reijonen et al., 2003; Wade et al., 2006). The lifetime prevalence rate for bulimia nervosa in a recent male and female adolescent sample was 0.9% (Swanson et al., 2011).

Binge eating disorder (BED) is more common than both anorexia nervosa and bulimia nervosa. It is estimated to occur in 3.5% of women and 2.0% of men at some point in their lifetime (Hudson et al., 2007). Wade and colleagues (2006) obtained similar results, estimating 2.9% lifetime prevalence for BED. Estimates for the prevalence of BED among adolescents range from 1.0% (Hoek & van Hoekn, 2003) to 1.6% (Swanson et al., 2011).

Feeding and eating conditions not elsewhere classified (formerly EDNOS) is an elusive category, and often accounts for greater numbers of diagnoses than the other eating disorders. Wade et al. (2006) estimated a 5.3% lifetime prevalence for EDNOS.

Onset and duration of these various eating disorders vary considerably. Onset of eating disorders is most common in adolescence, when approximately 10% of youth exhibit some symptoms of either AN or BN (Reijonen et al., 2003). Younger adolescents are most likely to exhibit symptoms of AN, while older adolescents are most likely to exhibit symptoms of BN (Hoek & van Hoeken, 2003; Reijonen et al., 2003). On average, individuals diagnosed with AN meet diagnostic criteria for only 1.7 years, while those diagnosed with BN and BED meet diagnostic criteria for an average of 8.3 and 8.1 years, respectively (Hudson et al., 2007).

Although relatively uncommon, eating disorders pose a significant public health concern due to their frequent comorbidity with other psychopathology and reported role impairment. Almost 95% of those with BN met diagnostic criteria for at least one other disorder in the *DSM-IV*, followed by 78.9% of those with BED and 56.2% of those with AN (Hudson et al., 2007). Significant comorbidity with common mood, anxiety, substance use, and impulse-control disorders have been reported by multiple researchers (Hudson et al., 2007; Reijonen et al., 2003). In addition to high comorbidity, the majority of those with eating disorders report role impairment in their home, work, personal, or social lives (Hudson et al., 2007).

To compound the problems of high comorbidity and role impairment, the majority of those with eating disorders do not seek treatment for their eating disorder (Hoek & van Hoeken, 2003). In one study, only 43.2% sought treatment for their BN, although they were slightly more likely to seek treatment for other conditions (Hudson et al., 2007). Similar results were reported for adolescents; most seek some form of treatment for a comorbid disorder, rather than the eating disorder (Swanson et al., 2011). Given that about 75% of women who seek treatment obtain a positive outcome (Wade et al., 2006), it is especially troubling that so many men and women are missing the opportunity to gain relief. Furthermore, the 10% mortality rate among those admitted to hospitals for the treatment of eating disorders indicates the grave consequences of failing to adequately identify and treat cases.

It is critical for researchers and clinicians to accurately identify those who meet diagnostic criteria for eating disorders in order to best help these clients. Although the majority of those who meet diagnostic criteria for eating disorders report role impairment, less than half seek treatment, making the identification of those with eating disorders a pressing concern for clinicians and researchers today.

HIGHLIGHTS OF FREE-ACCESS ASSESSMENTS USED TO IDENTIFY AND MONITOR OUTCOMES

There are various instruments available to assess eating disorder pathology in general or as it pertains to specific disorders. This section will highlight some of the most commonly used free-access instruments for the assessment of eating disorders.

Eating Attitudes Test

The first questionnaire developed to measure the symptoms of anorexia nervosa (Garner & Garfinkel, 1979), the Eating Attitudes Test (EAT) is now one of the most widely used self-report instruments for assessing eating disorders (Mintz & O'Halloran, 2000). The 40-item EAT was originally published in 1979 with a subsequent abbreviated revision published in 1982 (EAT-26). The EAT has been translated into seven languages and adapted for use with children. The EAT and EAT-26 are intended for use with adolescents and adults (Garner & Garfinkel, 1979). It is available, for free, at http://www.eat-26.com/index.htm.

The EAT is a Level A test, meaning that an advanced degree is not needed for administration, scoring, and interpretation. Administration of the EAT-26 takes approximately 15 minutes, and can be conducted either individually or in a group setting. The EAT-26 is composed of three parts. In Part A, the respondent is asked to provide demographic information, including height, weight, and age, which is later used to calculate Body Mass Index (BMI). Part B is composed of 26 Likert-type items on a six-point scale, with responses potentially ranging from 3 = "always" to 0 = "never." Part C includes five behavioral questions that ask respondents to indicate the frequency with which they engage in behaviors associated with eating disorders, such as binging and purging.

Scoring and interpretation varies for each part of the EAT-26. A formula is provided for calculating BMI from the information garnered in Part A. Each item on Part B receives three points for a response of "always," two points for a response of "usually," one point for a response of "often," and zero points for any other response. The lone exception is item 26, which is scored in the opposite direction. Although the 26 items compose three subscales (Dieting, Bulimia and Food Preoccupation, and Oral Control), item scores are simply summed to provide a total score on the EAT-26. For Part C, responses past the set behavioral threshold warrant concern. Immediate risk can be assessed by determining the frequency and context of affirmative behavioral responses.

Information from each part of the EAT-26 must be considered in interpretation. Garner (2011a) recommends pursuing a referral for professional evaluation of an eating disorder if a respondent meets any of the following three criteria: (a) an extremely underweight BMI according to age-matched population norms; (b) an EAT-26 total score of 20 or above; or (c) affirmative responses to any of the behavioral questions. While a score in excess of 20 shows a high level of concern regarding weight, dieting, and problematic eating behaviors, it does not necessarily indicate an eating disorder. The EAT-26 is thus inappropriate for diagnosis of an eating disorder, but is useful for screening and case-finding to identify individuals with an elevated risk of developing an eating disorder (Garner, 2011b).

Scores on the original EAT and the EAT-26 have been reported to be both reliable and valid. Garner and Garfinkel (1979) reported coefficient alphas of .79 for a group diagnosed with anorexia nervosa and .94 for a combined clinical and nonclinical population. Coefficient alphas of .90 for a group diagnosed with anorexia nervosa and .83 for a female comparison group were reported for scores on the EAT-26 (Garner, Olmstead, Bohr, & Garfinkel, 1982).

Criterion-related concurrent validity is evidenced by the correlation between total scores on the EAT and membership in the group diagnosed with anorexia nervosa (Garner & Garfinkel, 1979). Females with anorexia and comparison groups also have significantly different mean total scores (Garner et al., 1982). In regard to discriminant validity, the EAT is not significantly correlated with weight fluctuations, extraversion, or neuroticism. In regard to convergent validity, the EAT-26 is significantly correlated with body image, diet, and weight (Koslowsky et al., 1992). The EAT-26 is highly correlated with the EAT ($r = .98$), and scores on the EAT-26 provide a more efficient measure while their psychometric properties remain robust (Garner et al., 1982). Evidence for construct validity is provided by the factor analysis that identified three factors in the EAT-26. However, some researchers have failed to find evidence in support of the three-factor model and have instead proposed four- and five-factor models (Doninger, Enders, & Burnett, 2005; Koslowky et al., 1992; Ocker, Lam, Jensen, & Zhang, 2007). Koslowsky et al. suggested that the factor structure of the EAT-26 in nonclinical groups is different from that obtained in clinical groups.

The EAT-26 has both advantages and disadvantages. Given its economy in administration and scoring, the EAT-26 is an excellent screening measure for use in schools and athletic settings. Furthermore, the EAT-26 has a 90% accuracy rate when differentiating between those with and without eating disorders (Mintz & O'Halloran, 2000). The EAT-26 has been shown to be useful in identifying eating problems in nonclinical populations (Canals, Carbajo, & Fernandez-Ballart, 2002) and is sensitive to clinical remission (Garner & Garfinkel, 1979).

However, both versions of the EAT have a high false positive rate with nonclinical samples. Mintz and O'Halloran (2000) believe this to be a result of the monumental changes in criteria for the diagnosis of an eating disorder since the EAT and EAT-26 were originally developed. This highlights another problem with the EAT and EAT-26. Given that the EAT was developed to assess anorexia nervosa when bulimia was a symptom, rather than a separate diagnosis, many items on the EAT reflect bulimic symptoms - but it has not been validated as a measure of bulimia. Additionally, the EAT is inappropriate for use as the sole determinant of diagnosis and scores must be supplemented with clinical interviews and opinions (Garner, 2011b). Given its self-report format, the EAT is also susceptible to deception and denial by respondents. However, Garner reports that self-report instruments have been used successfully to screen for eating disorders. Finally, while BMI can provide skewed estimates of fatness for those who are athletic or from diverse ethnic groups, its effect is tempered since it is only one of three criteria that must be considered for referral (Garner, 2011a).

In conclusion, the EAT-26 is best used as a screening measure with nonclinical populations, such as in schools or athletic settings, or as an outcome measure with clinical populations (Garner et al., 1982). The multi-criteria scoring and interpretation approach of the EAT-26 provide diverse avenues for professionals to explore when making potential referrals. Overall, the EAT-26 is an efficient and well-researched instrument for assessing eating disorders in adolescents and adults.

SCOFF TEST

The SCOFF Test is a simple and fast screening tool used to detect the main symptoms of anorexia nervosa and bulimia nervosa (Morgan, Reid, & Lacey, 1999). The SCOFF can be used by non-specialists, and can even be self-administered in order to determine the potential need for referral to a mental health professional.

The SCOFF Test consists of five yes/no questions which assess purging, loss of control, weight loss, body image disturbance, and preoccupation with food. SCOFF is an acronym for a key feature assessed by each question. The questions are as follows: (a) Do you make yourself **Sick** because you feel uncomfortably full? (b) Do you worry you have lost **Control** over how much you eat? (c) Do you believe yourself to be fat when **Others** say you are too thin? (d) Have you recently lost more than **Fourteen** pounds in a three-month period? and (e) Would you say that **Food** dominates your life? One point is assigned for each "yes" answer, and these points are summed to obtain a total score. A total score of two or greater indicates a potential case of anorexia nervosa or bulimia nervosa.

Scores on the SCOFF Test have been reported to be both reliable and valid. Verbal and written versions demonstrated good agreement, with all five questions answered identically more than 90% of the time (Hill, Reid, Morgan, & Lacey, 2010). Perry et al. (2002) found good replicability between oral and written formats of the SCOFF as well, although higher scores were obtained when the written version was administered first and less consistency obtained when the interview came first, indicating that greater self-disclosure may be achieved by administering the SCOFF test in a written format. Scores on the SCOFF were associated with higher global and subscale scores on the EDE-Q (Parker, Lyons, & Bonner, 2005). Mond et al. (2008) also found the SCOFF to perform similarly to the EDE-Q. SCOFF scores also correlated strongly with EDI subscale scores (Hill et al., 2010) and total scores on the EAT-26 (Noma et al., 2006).

The SCOFF Test had high score sensitivity and specificity. Sensitivity is the proportion of individuals who have a diagnosable eating disorder that were accurately identified by the SCOFF (i.e., true positives), while specificity is the proportion of individuals who do not have a diagnosable eating disorder but were correctly identified by the SCOFF as not having an eating disorder (i.e., true negatives). Most reports of sensitivity for the SCOFF range from 72.0% to 100% (Cotton, Ball, & Robinson, 2003; Hill et al., 2010; Lähteenmäki et al., 2009; Mond et al., 2008; Morgan et al., 1999), although Parker et al. (2005) found that the SCOFF only identified half of those known to have an eating disorder. This low sensitivity may be due to the SCOFF's difficulty in identifying EDNOS individuals, since numerous researchers have reported on the SCOFF's near-perfect ability to identify those with AN and BN, but diminished capacity to identify individuals with EDNOS (Hill et al., 2010; Noma et al., 2006). Specificity estimates ranged from 73.0% to 93.2% (Cotton et al; Hill et al., 2010; Lähteenmäki et al., 2009; Mond et al., 2008; Morgan et al., 1999; Parker et al.).

The SCOFF is a psychometrically sound and efficient instrument for assessing potential eating disorder pathology. It is most appropriate for detecting the core features of anorexia nervosa and bulimia nervosa; it is more likely to miss cases of eating disorder not otherwise specified. However, given the fact that no significant differences in detection rates existed between the SCOFF and the EAT-26, a gold standard instrument in the assessment of eating disorders (Noma et al., 2006), the SCOFF is recommended as an excellent brief measure for determining likely cases of anorexia nervosa and bulimia nervosa for referral.

EATING DISORDER DIAGNOSTIC SCALE

The Eating Disorder Diagnostic Scale (EDDS) is a free-access instrument used to diagnose anorexia nervosa, bulimia nervosa, and binge eating disorder (Stice, Telch, & Rizvi, 2000). The EDDS is appropriate for use with adult women (Stice, Fisher, & Martinez, 2004), as well as male and female adolescents (Lee et al., 2007). It can be found online at http://homepage.psy.utexas.edu/homepage/group/sticelab/scales/.

The EDDS is composed of 22 items that address the diagnostic criteria for anorexia nervosa, bulimia nervosa, and binge eating disorder via a mixed format of dichotomous, frequency, Likert, and free response items. Computerized scoring algorithms are used to determine if individuals meet the diagnostic criteria for any of the possible eating disorders assessed (Stice et al., 2004), and can be obtained online at http://homepage.psy.utexas.edu/homepage/group/sticelab/scales/Images/SticeFisherMartinez04.pdf. Hand scoring for each item is also possible by following the directions (Stice, Telch, and Rizvi, 2000) provided online at http://homepage.psy.utexas.edu/homepage/group/sticelab/scales/Images/SticeTelch00.pdf.

Scores on the EDDS have strong evidence of reliability. Stice et al. (2000) reported test-retest reliability of .87. Lee et al. (2007) obtained poor test-retest reliability for diagnoses over a one-month period, which may be because behavioral items are less consistent than cognitive items. Internal consistency coefficients of .89 have been obtained by multiple researchers (Stice et al., 2000; Stice et al., 2004). A sensitivity of .88 and a specificity of .98 have been reported for the overall measure (Stice et al., 2004), while sensitivities range from .77 to .93 and specificities range from .96 to 1.00 for each eating disorder (Stice et al., 2000). Thus, the EDDS demonstrates a high accuracy rate when identifying individuals with anorexia nervosa, and a slightly less strong, but still high, accuracy rate when identifying individuals with bulimia nervosa and binge eating disorder respectively. In addition, the consistently high measures of specificity result in a very low false positive rate, rendering the EDDS both cost-effective and sensitive to true cases of eating disorders.

Strong evidence of the validity of EDDS scores has been published as well. Experts on eating disorders have established content validity for the EDDS (Stice et al., 2000). Numerous researchers have demonstrated the convergent validity of the EDDS via its high correlations with other scales purported to measure eating disorders, including the EDE-Q, a highly respected instrument (Lee et al., 2007; Stice et al., 2000; Stice et al., 2004). Criterion validity has been established with high agreement between EDDS scores and interview-based diagnoses (Stice et al., 2000; Stice et al., 2004). Predictive validity is evident due to the ability of scores on the EDDS to predict response to a prevention program, as well as future onset of eating pathology and depression (Stice et al., 2004). Lee and colleagues (2007) found evidence of a four-factor structure in the EDDS, with acceptable internal consistency coefficients for all of these factors.

Overall, the EDDS is a useful instrument for diagnosing anorexia nervosa, bulimia nervosa, and binge eating disorder. Reliability and validity of EDDS scores have both been intensively researched and well established. Slightly lower than expected test-retest reliabilities for diagnoses are in keeping with the finding that the behaviors associated with bulimia nervosa and binge eating disorder are not necessarily stable over time (Lee et al., 2007). The sensitivity of the EDDS in detecting intervention effects (Stice et al., 2004) suggest that this instrument could be valuable in demonstrating the effectiveness of various counseling interventions. Those who decide to use the EDDS are cautioned to avoid making diagnoses without extensive clinical training and triangulation of information, and should instead use EDDS scores as an initial starting point for referrals, or additional information gathering.

BODY SHAPE QUESTIONNAIRE

The Body Shape Questionnaire (BSQ) was developed to measure concerns about body shape, since body image disturbance is a common feature of eating disorders (Cooper, Taylor, Cooper, & Fairburn, 1987). Notably, the BSQ has been translated and validated in both Swedish (Ghaderi & Scott, 2004) and French (Rousseau, Knotter, Barbe, Raich, & Chabrol, 2005). Numerous abbreviated versions of the BSQ have been developed for efficiency and clinical utility, including multiple eight, 10, and 16-item versions (Evans & Dolan, 1993; Mazzeo, 1999). The BSQ is appropriate for use with adult females. Various forms of the BSQ are available at http://www.psyctc.org/tools/bsq/.

The BSQ is a Level B instrument. Thus, the administrator must either be, or be supervised by, a clinician or researcher in the mental health field. Completion of the BSQ requires approximately 10 minutes. The BSQ is a self-report instrument composed of 34 Likert-type items scored on a six-point scale ranging from "never" to "always" (Cooper et al., 1987). A total score is obtained by summing responses on all of the items. Total scores on the BSQ range from 34 to 204, with higher scores indicating greater concern with body shape.

Sufficient score reliability data have been reported. Cooper et al. (1987) failed to report reliability coefficients in their publication regarding the development of the BSQ, but Evans and Dolan (1993) reported a coefficient alpha of .97 and satisfactory inter-item correlations for BSQ scores from a nonclinical population. Rosen, Jones, Ramirez, and Waxman (1996) have reported a test-retest reliability coefficient of .88. Abbreviated and translated versions of the BSQ have also been reported to have high reliability estimates (Evans & Dolan, 1993; Ghaderi & Scott, 2004; Mazzeo, 1999).

Scores on the BSQ indicated adequate degrees of score validity. Scores on the BSQ correlated moderately with scores on the EAT and on the Body Dissatisfaction subscale of the EDI for bulimia nervosa patients (Cooper et al., 1987). Scores on the BSQ correlated highly with scores on the EAT for a female comparison group. Obtained mean scores for probable bulimics in the community did not differ from obtained mean scores for diagnosed bulimics. As would be expected, BSQ scores did significantly differ for female comparisons and those seeking treatment or therapy for obesity or body image disturbances (Rosen et al., 1996). Other researchers also established criterion-based concurrent validity as evidenced by moderate to high correlations with similar measures of concern with appearance for clinical and nonclinical samples (Evans & Dolan, 1993; Ghaderi & Scott, 2004; Mazzeo, 1999; Rosen et al., 1996). Discriminant validity is evidenced by the low correlation of scores on the BSQ with scores on measures of anxiety and depression (Evans & Dolan, 1993). In support of construct validity, factor analysis has supported a unidimensional model (Evans & Dolan, 1993; Mazzeo, 1999).

The BSQ has both advantages and disadvantages. Simple and brief, it has sound efficiency and clinical utility in both its full and abbreviated versions. Mazzeo (1999) has suggested that the BSQ would be a useful screening device for assessing excessive concern with body shape in undergraduates. However, interpreters must be careful not to extrapolate scores on the BSQ to assume additional symptoms or diagnosis of an eating disorder. Unfortunately, insufficient data regarding the use of the BSQ with men has been published, rendering the BSQ inappropriate for use with men at this time. Fortunately, Rosen et al. (1996) have begun the process of validating the BSQ for use with men. Additionally, use of some of the eight-item abbreviated versions of the BSQ may be trading practicality for sound psychometrics. Although they were highly correlated with each other, some versions were statistically different from other versions, and the validation sample had poor confirmatory factor analysis results (Evans & Dolan, 1993). Furthermore, Mazzeo (1999) calls attention to the fact that Evans and Dolan failed to cross-validate their results on a new sample, which could lead to spuriously strong psychometrics.

In summary, the BSQ is an easy and efficient way to assess concerns regarding body shape. Because body image disturbance is a central feature of eating disorders, the BSQ can provide insight into this facet of eating disorders in clinical populations. Although Mazzeo (1999) suggested the potential usefulness of the BSQ as a screening measure for preoccupation with body image, the BSQ was originally recommended for use as a measure of the extent of concerns about body shape, rather than as an instrument for detecting cases of eating disorders (Cooper et al., 1987). It seems that the BSQ is best suited for gathering information regarding body image disturbance in both clinical and nonclinical populations.

Because body image disturbance is related to the development and treatment outcomes of eating disorders (Mazzeo, 1999), this information could prove invaluable in referral and treatment options.

BULIMIC INVESTIGATORY TEST, EDINBURGH

The Bulimic Investigatory Test, Edinburgh (BITE), is a self-report inventory used to identify those with symptoms of binge eating or bulimia, which are deemed synonymous here. While the BITE was designed for use as a screening instrument to identify those who display the symptoms of binge eating, the BITE can also serve as a useful measure of severity and progress in treatment (Henderson & Freeman, 1987).

An optional demographic and general data sheet relevant to the study and treatment of binge eating precedes the BITE. The BITE itself contains 33 items, 30 of which compose the symptom scale, while the remaining three items make up the severity scale. The items on the symptom scale are all dichotomous questions to which the client is asked to respond "yes" or "no." The items on the severity scale use a Likert-type format to assess the frequency of various behaviors associated with bulimia (ie., fasting, taking laxatives, bingeing). For example, item 27 asks respondents to rate how often they binge on a 1–6 point scale (1 = hardly ever; 2 = once a month; 3 = once a week; 4 = 2–3 times a week; 5 = daily; 6 = 2–3 times a day). Completion of the BITE takes approximately 10 minutes. It can be administered in a group or individual setting.

For the symptom scale, all questions score one point for a "yes" response, with the exception of the five items in which a "no" response indicates disordered eating attitudes or behaviors – these five items receive one point each for a "no" response. All 30 questions on the symptom scale are summed; thus, scores on the symptom scale can range from 0 to 30. Henderson and Freeman (1987) suggested that a symptom score in excess of 20 indicates a highly disordered eating pattern and a high likelihood that the client will fulfill diagnostic criteria for bulimia. Those who score between 10 and 19 have an unusual, subclinical eating pattern; Henderson and Freeman urged practitioners to follow up scores ranging from 15 to 19 with an interview. Those who score below 10 are considered normal.

Administrators simply sum the numbers corresponding to the circled responses for the three questions that comprise the severity scale, which are items 6, 7, and 27. Scores on the severity scale can range from two to 39. A score of five or more on the severity scale is deemed clinically significant, while a score of 10 or more displays a high degree of severity, as defined by frequency of bingeing and purging behavior. Regardless of the symptom score, Henderson and Freeman (1987) recommend that any score equal to, or in excess of, five be followed up by an interview.

Scores on the BITE have been found to have adequate reliability and validity. Henderson and Freeman (1987) reported internal consistency coefficients of .96 for the symptom scale and .62 for the severity scale. Fonseca-Pedrero, Sierra-Baigrie, Paino, Lemos-Giráldez, and Muñiz (2011) reported similar internal consistency coefficients of .95 for the Symptom scale and .70 for the Severity scale. Test-retest reliability was .86 for non-bulimic women and .68 for bulimic women (Henderson & Freeman, 1987). Subsequent international studies have reported very similar results (Fonseca-Pedrero et al., 2011). The BITE correlates moderately with the total Eating Attitudes Test (EAT) total score, as well as its diet and binge subscales. It also correlates moderately with the binge eating and "drive to thinness" subscales on the Eating Disorders Inventory (EDI) (Henderson & Freeman, 1987). Fonseca-Pedrero et al. (2011) have confirmed that the current one-factor model of the BITE fits the data adequately.

Overall, the BITE is useful due to its brevity and specificity for binge eating behaviors. By allowing for a subclinical range of scores, the BITE is successful in detecting cases of disordered eating that are not severe enough to warrant a clinical score, but which are still markedly different from what are considered normal eating attitudes and patterns. It is appropriate for use with adolescent males and females, as well as young adult females. However, the BITE is not necessarily appropriate for detecting binge eaters of a low weight, or differentiating among eating disorders. Finally, it may distort the extent of respondent pathology due to its mainly dichotomous nature.

Bulimia Test—Revised

The Bulimia Test (BULIT) was designed to assess the symptoms of bulimia nervosa, primarily for use in screening nonclinical populations (Smith & Thelen, 1984). Originally based on the *DSM-III* criteria, subsequent revisions of the *DSM* have resulted in further revision of the BULIT (BULIT-R; Thelen, Farmer, Wonderlich, & Smith, 1991) and continued validation efforts to ensure that the BULIT still adequately assesses the diagnostic criteria put forth in the most recent editions of the *DSM* (Thelen, Mintz, & Vander Wal, 1996). The BULIT-R is appropriate for use with female adolescents and adults (McCarthy, Simmons, Smith, Tomlinson, & Hill, 2002). It is also appropriate for use with various ethnic groups (Fernandez, Malacrne, Wilfley, & McQuaid, 2006) and translations have been validated for use in Spain (Bernos-Hernandez et al., 2007) and Korea (Ryu, Lyle, Galer-Unti, & Black, 1999). It can be accessed via the original article publication.

The BULIT-R is composed of 28 items that assess the symptoms of bulimia nervosa scored on a five-point Likert scale, as well as eight unscored items related to weight control behavior. All responses are summed to obtain a total score (Smith & Thelen, 1984). Thelen and colleagues (1991) recommend that scores equal to, or in excess of, 104 indicate the presence of bulimia.

Scores on the BULIT-R have been reported to be highly reliable and moderately valid. Test-retest reliabilities for the BULIT and BULIT-R range from .87 to .95 in nonclinical and symptomatic populations (Brelsford, Hummel, & Barrios, 1992; Smith & Thelen, 1984; Thelen et al., 1991). Internal consistency coefficients have consistently exceeded .90 (Bernos-Hernandez et al, 2007; Brelsford et al., 1992; Fernandez et al., 2006; McCarthy et al., 2002; Ryu et al., 1999; Thelen et al., 1996). Scores on the BULIT and BULIT-R significantly differentiated between those with bulimia nervosa and controls (Smith & Thelen, 1984; Thelen et al, 1991; Thelen et al., 1996). In support of convergent validity, the BULIT and BULIT-R correlated moderately to highly with the Binge Scale, the EAT, most subscales of the EDI-2, and self-report diary measures of bingeing and purging (Brelsford et al., 1992; McCarthy et al, 2002; Ryu et al, 1999; Smith & Thelen, 1984; Thelen et al., 1991). The specificity of the BULIT-R is .96, while measures of sensitivity range from .62 (Thelen et al., 1991) to .91 (Thelen et al., 1996). Evidence for construct validity via factor analysis is shaky. Although Smith and Thelen originally identified a seven-factor structure in the BULIT, Thelen and colleagues found a five-factor structure in the BULIT-R. Subsequent researchers have found four- and six-factor models to better fit different ethnic groups

(Bernos-Hernadez et al., 2007; Fernandez et al., 2006). McCarthy and colleagues (2002) found a one-factor model to be the best fit for adolescent scores.

The BULIT-R is an efficient and inexpensive measure of the symptoms of bulimia. It is likely best used as a screening measure in nonclinical populations. However, the inconsistency of its factor structure has caused some to question its ability to adequately measure a stable multifaceted construct (Bernos-Hernandez et al., 2007).

THREE-FACTOR EATING QUESTIONNAIRE

The Three-Factor Eating Questionnaire (TFEQ) was originally published to measure eating behaviors, specifically along the dimensions of dietary restraint, disinhibition, and hunger (Stunkard & Messick, 1985). The TFEQ is also known as the Eating Inventory (EI). Numerous researchers have adapted and modified the original TFEQ for their own purposes, resulting in various abbreviated versions of the TFEQ with psychometric properties similar to the original TFEQ (Cappelleri et al., 2009; Karlsson, Persson, Sjöström, & Sullivan, 2000; Tholin, Rasmussen, Tynelius, & Karlsson, 2005). The TFEQ is appropriate for use with both men and women over the age of 17 years, and is available in the literature via the original publication.

The TFEQ is composed of 51 items, which are representative of three domains: dietary restraint (R), disinhibition (D), and hunger (H). The first 36 items, comprising Part I, are dichotomous true-false items. The 15 items comprising Part II are Likert-type items with varying possible response choices (i.e., 1 = rarely; 2 = sometimes; 3 = usually; 4 = always). Item 50 is an exception, providing respondents with six possible response choices. Administration of the TFEQ takes approximately 15 minutes, and can be conducted either individually or in groups (Haynes, 1998).

An answer sheet is provided for scoring. One point is given for each designated true or false in Part I. In Part II, each question is bisected either positively or negatively. Responses on the designated side of the split are given one point. Thus, although respondents are given more options from which to choose, their answers are scored dichotomously to mirror the scoring methodology of Part I. The answer key indicates which domain each item assesses, and all items comprising each domain are summed to determine a total score for each of the three subscales, which results in a possible 0–51 point total score.

Directions and tables are provided to aid administrators in determining how examinee scores compare with normal and obese populations (Bloom, 1998). Although a table of normative guidelines for interpreting raw scores is presented, the manual exhorts the importance of professional judgment in score interpretation, due to the paucity of available normative data. The manual suggests that interpretation should be supplemented with clinical interviews and observations (Haynes, 1998). Elevated scores on the cognitive restraint scale are considered positive, while elevated scores on the disinhibition and hunger scales are considered negative. While substantially high or low scores on one or more factors can be useful in planning treatment, it is important to note that strict cognitive restraint may be problematic for those battling eating disorders.

Scores on the TFEQ have been found to be reliable. Stunkard and Messick (1985) cited coefficient alphas of .93 for dietary restraint, .91 for disinhibition, and .85 for hunger for a combined group of free and restrained eaters. Shearin, Russ, Hull, Clarkin, and Smith (1994) found scores on the TFEQ to have an overall coefficient alpha of .91. Test-retest reliability coefficients were reported to be high, all exceeding .80 (Stunkard & Messick). However, given that these coefficients were obtained from an unpublished study using a small sample, further evidence of test-retest reliability is warranted. Partial evidence has been provided by reports of test-retest reliability for the restraint scale as .91 (Allison, Kalinsky, & Gorman, 1992).

While some evidence exists for the validity of scores on the TFEQ, gaps remain. In support of content validity, Stunkard and Messick (1985) report using an extensive literature review and refinement process in item construction and selection. Criterion-related validity is supported by the findings that reports of both binge severity and overeating during a laboratory study correlated with scores on the disinhibition subscale. Moderate to high correlations also existed between various related subscales on the TFEQ and the EAT, EDI, and BULIT (Shearin et al., 1994). Additionally, scores on the TFEQ restraint scale are strongly inversely correlated with caloric intake (Allison et al., 1992). Thus there appears to be evidence of convergent and discriminant validity in support of construct validity. However, the construct validity of the TFEQ has been questioned by those who have failed to replicate the proposed three-factor structure of the TFEQ (Mazzeo, Aggen, Anderson, Tozzi, & Bulik, 2003).

Overall, the TFEQ is an efficient and easily administered instrument used to assess eating behaviors. It is most appropriate for use in gathering data to inform treatment planning and evaluation (Bloom, 1998). The lack of normative data makes interpretation more difficult and less reliable. Scores on the TFEQ are not sufficient to make a diagnosis, and must be supplanted with clinical observation and judgment.

Binge Eating Scale

The Binge Eating Scale (BES) is a free online instrument that assesses behavioral, emotional, and cognitive components associated with binge eating (Gormally, Black, Daston, & Rardin, 1982). It is used to assess binge eating in obese individuals, and is able to discriminate among individuals judged to have various severities of binge eating problems. It can be accessed online at http://psychology-tools.com/binge-eating-scale/.

The BES is composed of 16 polytomous items. Each item has three or four potential responses, each of which increases in severity or intensity. The least symptomatic response is scored as a zero, with each successive response receiving one, two, or three points. The maximum score on the BES is 47. Scores are interpreted based on a cut-off method (Celio, Wilfley, Crow, Mitchell, & Walsh, 2004). Scores greater than, or equal to, 27 indicate severe binge eating, while scores between 17 and 27 indicate moderate binge eating. Scores below 17 indicate mild or no binge eating.

There is little evidence for the reliability and validity of BES scores. Timmerman (1999) found moderate correlations between BES scores and the severity of binge eating episodes as assessed by food diaries. However, BES scores were not related to total caloric intake and were unable to distinguish between subjective and objective binge eating. Celio et al. (2004) similarly found that BES scores were correlated with objective binge episode frequency and days, but not with subjective binge episodes. The BES had good sensitivity at .85, but extremely poor specificity at .20. Thus, the BES would likely result in high number of false positives, making this instrument potentially excessively time consuming and expensive.

Although the BES can provide some information about the severity of binges in obese individuals, its lack of appropriate reliability and validity evidence render it a questionable choice for assessing binge eating. These problems are likely due in part to the fact that the BES was designed before binge eating disorder was conceptualized. The BES is likely best used as a screen for the detection of binge eating.

SHORT EVALUATION OF EATING DISORDERS

Developed by Bauer, Winn, Schmidt, and Kordy (2005), the Short Evaluation of Eating Disorders (SEED) was designed to assess the major symptoms of anorexia nervosa and bulimia nervosa in a simple, six-item format. Administration requires only five minutes.

Three items each are devoted to the assessment of anorexia nervosa and bulimia nervosa. Items are presented in mixed behavioral frequency, Likert-type, and dichotomous formats. Symptoms are rated from zero to three, with higher scores indicating greater severity. As the most prominent symptoms of their respective disorders, the items assessing the respondent's degree of overweight and amount of binge eating count for twice as much in scoring. Items corresponding to anorexia nervosa and bulimia nervosa are summed separately and divided by four to yield a severity index. Cut-off scores have yet to be proposed.

Initial evidence for the reliability and validity of SEED scores is promising, but more evidence is necessary. Bauer et al. (2005) obtained low to moderate correlations between SEED scores and EDI susbscale and total scores. Criterion validity is evidenced by the fact that most items accurately discriminated between those with anorexia nervosa, those with bulimia nervosa, and controls. The high level of agreement between patients' and clinicians' overall ratings provided a measure of concurrent validity.

The SEED appears to be an efficient and useful instrument in assessing the major symptoms of anorexia nervosa and bulimia nervosa. However, its reliability and cut-off score usefulness for those with EDNOS have yet to be assessed. The SEED may be useful as a screening test, but more information is needed regarding its psychometrics.

Rating of Anorexia and Bulimia Interview

The Rating of Anorexia and Bulimia Interview (RABI) assesses symptoms of eating disorders, related psychopathology, and background variables pertinent to those diagnosed with eating disorders (Clinton & Norring, 1999). It is available, free of charge, online at http://www.atstorning.se/documents/BAB_article.pdf, but is limited to use by mental health professionals with a master's degree and graduate training in tests and measurement.

The semi-structured interview is composed of 56 items, which comprise four subscales, including body shape and weight preoccupation, binge eating, anorexic eating behavior, and compensatory behavior (Clinton & Norring, 1999). Items are scaled on a Likert-type scale with three to five points. A revised version, created by Nevonen, Broberg, Clinton, and Norring (2003) consists of 36 items with six subscales, including anorexic eating behavior, body shape and preoccupation, bulimic symptoms, partner relationships, parental relationships, and peer relationships. Of these items, 34 are grouped on relevant clinical problem areas, including co-occurring problems, compensatory behavior, treatment, concomitant problems, and treatment motivation.

Little evidence of score reliability and validity was gathered. Coefficient alphas of .87 for the anorexia index and .82 for the bulimia index were reported by Clinton and Norring (1999). Subsequent researchers obtained subscale coefficient alphas ranging from .71 to .86, with the exception of anorexia eating behavior (.42) and peer relationships (.63) (Nevonen et al., 2003). Nevonen and colleagues obtained unacceptably low test-retest coefficients for anorexic behavior, compensatory behavior, and peer relationships. Clinton and Norring found only low to moderate correlations between RABI scores and scores on the EDI subscales, but Nevonen and colleagues found moderate to high correlations with the EDI when using their revised version of the RABI. Prediction of *DSM* eating disorders using the RABI is poor (Clinton & Norring).

Adequate evidence of reliability and validity thus remain to be established with the RABI. While the RABI has been used to determine potential diagnoses, it is probably currently most appropriate for use as a screening measure.

VARIOUS ADDITIONAL ONLINE MEASURES

A plethora of other measures of eating disorder assessment exist online for free. The majority of these tests are designed to be self-administered. The following is a list of assessments composed of dichotomous and Likert-type items for which there is not yet any existing psychometric data to support their use. They may be helpful for educational or conversational purposes.

- BL:Eating Disorders Assessment Test (12 yes/no item screen for detecting symptoms of anorexia and bulimia): http://www.healthyplace.com/psychological-tests/eating-disorders-assessment-test/.
- Eating Disorder Quiz (22-item true/false and 4-point Likert-type questions to detect tendencies toward anorexia or bulimia): http://www.casapalmera.com/assessments/eating-disorder-self-assessment.php
- Eating Disorder Test (22-item 4-point Likert-type questions to detect a potential eating disorder): http://www.caringonline.com/eatdis/misc/edtest.htm.
- Adolescent Eating Disorder Screen (11 yes/no item eating disorder screen): http://www.mha-oc.org/EDtest1.html.
- Do I Have an Eating Disorder? (20 4-point Likert-type items to detect probably eating disorders): http://www.netdoctor.co.uk/interactive/interactivetests/eatingdisorder.php.
- Online Eating Disorder Evaluation (37 yes/no item screen for detecting eating disorder symptoms): http://www.mirasol.net/ed-recovery/assessments/online-evaluation.php.

Chapter 8

Assessment of Trauma and Stressor-Related Disorders

Trauma and Stressor-Related Disorders Commonly Encountered in Clinical Practice

Most people will be exposed to traumatic stress at least once in their lifetime (Ozer, Best, Lipsey, & Weiss, 2008). Examples of potentially traumatic stressors include, but are not limited to, the loss of a loved one, serious illness, motor vehicle accidents, natural disasters, terrorist attacks, and being a witness to or victim of any type of abuse. Thus, the majority of the disorders that comprise the *DSM-5* category "Trauma and Stressor-Related Disorders" are well known to both the general public and the mental health community. Fortunately, the prominence of these disorders in the general population has prompted extensive research into etiology, symptom dimensions, and treatment.

Disorders in the "Trauma and Stressor-Related Disorders" category include reactive attachment disorder, disinhibited social engagement disorder, acute stress disorder, posttraumatic stress disorder, adjustment disorders, and trauma or stressor-related disorder not elsewhere classified (APA, 2013). Because clinicians are most likely to encounter acute stress disorder, posttraumatic stress disorder, and adjustment disorders, these disorders will be the focus of the present chapter. Persistent complex bereavement disorder will also be highlighted, as it is a new disorder in the *DSM-5*.

ACUTE STRESS DISORDER AND POSTTRAUMATIC STRESS DISORDER

Acute stress disorder (ASD) is characterized by the development of intrusion, dissociation, avoidance, and arousal symptoms in response to a traumatic event (APA, 2013). Criterion A requires that an individual must have been exposed to an actual or threatened death, serious injury, or sexual violation, either by directly experiencing the event, witnessing the event, learning that the event happened to a close family member or friend, or experiencing repeated or extreme exposure to aversive details of the traumatic event, with the exclusion of media exposure. In order to meet Criterion B, an individual must present with at least nine symptoms in the following four categories: (a) intrusion, (b) dissociative, (c) avoidance, and (d) arousal. Intrusion symptoms include the following: (a) distressing memories of the event, (b) distressing dreams, (c) dissociative reactions, and (d) psychological distress related to the traumatic event. Dissociation symptoms include: (a) unable to express positive feelings, (b) feelings of unreality, and (c) unable to remember important details from the event. Avoidance symptoms include efforts to avoid the following: (a) distressing memories, thoughts, or feelings about the event, and (b) external reminders of the event. Arousal symptoms include: (a) disturbance of normal sleeping patterns, (b) irritableness or aggressiveness, (c) hypervigilance, (d) unable to concentrate, and (e) easily startled. The disturbance must occur for three days to one month after the exposure to trauma and cause clinically significant distress or impairment in social, occupational, or other important areas of functioning. Finally, the disturbance cannot better be explained by the criteria for brief psychotic disorder, or be due to the direct effects of a substance or another medical condition. Severity is evaluated using a five-point Likert-type scale that assesses the extent of seven key symptoms.

The criteria required for a diagnosis of posttraumatic stress disorder (PTSD) are strikingly similar to the criteria required for a diagnosis of acute stress disorder, but are marked by greater severity and duration of symptoms (APA, 2013). Criterion A for PTSD is identical to Criterion A for ASD. Criterion B requires that an individual present with at least one of the intrusion symptoms, which are identical to the intrusion symptoms listed for ASD with the addition of marked physiological reactions to reminders of the traumatic event. In order to meet Criterion

C, individuals must present with at least one of the avoidance symptoms outlined in ASD. Criterion D requires that individuals experience negative changes in cognitions and mood as evidenced by at least two of the following: (a) poor memory of the event, (b) negative beliefs about self or others, (c) self-blame or blaming others about the event's cause or consequences, (d) negative emotionality, (e) lack of interest in life activities, (f) detached feelings, and (g) unable to express positive feeling. Criterion E requires that individuals experience significant changes in arousal and reactivity associated with the traumatic event, as evidenced by at least two of the following: (a) irritability or aggressiveness, (b) recklessness or self-destructiveness, (c) hypervigilance, (d) easily startled, (e) concentration problems, and (f) disturbance of normal sleep patterns. The duration of the disturbance must be greater than one month, and it must cause clinically significant distress or impairment in social, occupational,, or other important areas of functioning. Finally, the disturbance cannot better be explained by the direct effects of a substance or another medical condition. Clinicians must specify "PTSD with delayed expression" if the diagnostic criteria are not met for at least six months after the event. Two subtypes, "PTSD in preschool children" and "PTSD with prominent dissociate symptoms," are also included under the PTSD diagnosis with additional qualifiers. Severity is evaluated using a five-point Likert-type scale that assesses the extent of seven key symptoms.

Given the substantial degree of overlap among ASD and PTSD symptoms, many have examined the utility of ASD diagnoses as a predictor for later PTSD diagnoses. While some promote the predictive value of ASD diagnoses (Brewin, Andrews, Rose, & Kirk, 1999; Kangas, Henry, & Bryant, 2005; Meiser-Stedman, Yule, Smith, Glucksman, & Dalgleish, 2005), most have found that ASD diagnoses are a poor screener for the identification of children and adults who eventually develop PTSD (Bryant, 2011; Bryant, Salmon, Sinclair, & Davidson, 2007; Creamer, O'Donnell, & Pattison, 2004). Creamer et al. suggested that re-experiencing and arousal symptoms in ASD are more accurate predictors of later PTSD. Although most people with an ASD diagnosis eventually develop some type of psychiatric disorder, the majority of people who eventually met criteria for PTSD did not initially meet criteria for ASD (Bryant, Creamer, O'Donnell, Silove, & McFarlane, 2012). Thus, while

ASD diagnoses pose a risk factor for psychiatric disorders in general, they fail to adequately predict the later development of PTSD.

Although approximately 50–60% of the U.S. population is at some point exposed to traumatic stress, only 5–10% developed PTSD (Ozer et al., 2008). Thus, researchers have sought to determine what makes those individuals who develop PTSD different to those who do not develop PTSD. Although ASD diagnoses did not prove to be a valuable predictor of PTSD, many other risk factors have been identified. An individual's psychological resiliency and meaning-making of the traumatic event are the strongest predictors of who will develop PTSD, although adjustment, prior exposure to trauma, posttrauma social support, and concurrent psychopathology play important roles as well. Overall, the way an individual responds after a trauma carries substantially more predictive power than pre-existing characteristics in predicting PTSD in children, adolescents, and adults (Ozer et al., 2008; Trickey, Siddaway, Meiser-Stedman, Serpell, & Field, 2012). Similar results have been obtained in the prediction of ASD development (Fugslang, Moergeli, Hepp-Beg, & Schnyder, 2002).

Despite the fact that posttrauma factors possess greater predictive power, certain demographic characteristics have also been identified as risk factors for PTSD. Groups at increased risk for developing PTSD following a traumatic event include females, Caucasians, African-Americans, immigrants, refugees, and deployed members of the military (Israelski et al., 2007; Magruder & Yeager, 2009; Ozer et al., 2008; Tolin & Foa, 2008).

The lifetime prevalence estimates of PTSD in the general population range from 7.4% to 12.3% (Beck & Coffey, 2007; Ozer et al., 2008), but prevalence estimates in populations exposed to specific significant traumas are much higher. Of parents of hospitalized infants, 11.5% (Lefkowitz, Baxt, & Evans, 2010) later developed PTSD, as did 22.8% of parents of children with chronic illnesses (Cabizuca, Marques-Portella, Mendlowicz, Coutinho, & Figueira, 2009). In addition, 34% of HIV-infected primary care patients (Israelski et al., 2007), 14% of individuals who received a cancer diagnosis (Kangas et al., 2005), 17.5–42% of people who experienced a serious injury (O'Donnell, Creamer, Bryant, Schnyder, & Shalev, 2003), 39% of women who experienced a first-trimester miscarriage (Bowles et al., 2006), and 25–33% of individuals involved in a motor vehicle accident (Beck & Coffey, 2007) later developed PTSD. Furthermore, 20% of victims of violent crime (Brewin et al., 1999), 46.2% of those in an impoverished urban population (Gillespie et al., 2009), and 2–17% of those in the military, affected by factors such as combat role and cultural background (Creamer, Wade, Fletcher, & Forbes, 2011), later developed PTSD. ASD is also more prevalent in these populations, with 29.5% of parents of infants hospitalized in NICU (Lefkowitz et al., 2010), 43% of HIV-infected primary care patients (Israelski et al., 2007), 28% of women who experienced a first-trimester miscarriage (Bowles et al., 2006), 19.4% of children and adolescents involved in assaults or car accidents (Mesier-Stedman et al., 2005), and 19% of victims of violent crime (Brewin et al., 1999) developing ASD. Incredibly, 75% of gunshot-injured youth displayed ASD symptoms, as compared to 14% of medically ill youth (Hamrin & Scahill, 2004). ASD and PTSD are clearly pressing problems on the mental health agenda today.

Fortunately, numerous researchers have sought to determine the most efficacious treatments for PTSD, and have obtained promising, consistent results. The most recent evidence points to the overwhelming superiority of trauma-focused cognitive-behavioral therapy (CBT) and eye movement desensitization and reprocessing (EMDR) as the most efficacious treatments for PTSD for both children and adults (Ehlers et al., 2010; Ponniah & Hollon, 2009; Roberts, Kitchiner, Kenardy, & Bisson, 2009). School-based interventions, such as CBT, play and art therapies, EMDR, and mind-body techniques, have also been shown to be highly effective in reducing PTSD symptoms in children and adolescents (Rolfsnes & Idsoe, 2011).

In order to provide optimal treatment, clinicians must accurately differentiate ASD and PTSD symptoms from those of depression, anxiety, and substance use disorders, which are frequently comorbid with disorders in the Trauma and Stressor-Related Disorders category (Beck & Coffey, 2007; Creamer et al., 2011; Israelski et al., 2007; Kangas et al., 2005). Therefore, it is of critical importance that clinicians use the best available instruments for screening, assessment, and diagnosis of ASD and PTSD, in order to accurately identify and treat this substantial population.

Adjustment Disorders

Adjustment Disorders, or the development of clinically significant emotional or behavioral symptoms, occur in some individuals as a response to a stressor (APA, 2013). Criterion A requires that the onset of symptoms must occur within three months of the onset of the stressor, and Criterion B requires that the symptoms must be evidenced by at least one of the following: (a) excessive distress disproportionate to the stressor, and (b) substantial social, occupational, or other functional impairment. In addition, the disturbance cannot be better explained by another mental disorder or as an exacerbation of a pre-existing mental disorder. Once the stressor, or its consequences, has ended, the symptoms do not persist for longer than six months, with the exception of the "related to bereavement" subtype. The clinician must specify one of the following subtypes based on the most predominant symptom: (a) with depressed mood, (b) with anxiety, (c) with mixed anxiety and depressed mood, (d) with disturbance of conduct, (e) with mixed disturbance of emotions and conduct, (f) with features of acute stress disorder or post-traumatic stress disorder, (g) related to bereavement, or (h) unspecified. Additional qualifiers apply to the "related to bereavement" subtype.

Currently, there is a dearth of information in the literature regarding the prevalence and treatment of adjustment disorders. Casey and Doherty (2012) suggest that adjustment disorders are under-researched due to the problems presented by the lack of specificity in their diagnostic criteria. Because researchers have neglected to enhance their understanding of how best to identify and treat adjustment disorders, no screening or assessment instruments specific to them currently exist. Current screening instruments are unable to effectively differentiate adjustment disorders from major depressive disorder, and most commonly-used clinical interviews fail to include the adjustment disorders diagnosis altogether.

Although adjustment disorders are typically short-term, and often go away without treatment (Casey & Doherty, 2012), it is imperative for clinicians to enhance their screening capabilities for adjustment disorders. The typically short duration of the disorder does not negate the importance of alleviating the troubling effects on the quality of life. Furthermore, severe cases are associated with heightened suicide risk, so allowing these cases to go unrecognized and untreated could have potentially disastrous consequences. It seems that the best available treatment for adjustment disorders is brief psychotherapy with a focus on the specific subtype of each individual client. Evidence for the use of medications is currently lacking.

Future researchers are charged with the critically important task of designing screening instruments specific to adjustment disorders, or enhancing current screening instruments of mood, anxiety, and conduct disorders, in order to effectively differentiate subtypes of adjustment disorders from these other mental disorders. The small amount of prevalence data available indicates that adjustment disorders likely affect 11–18% of individuals in primary care settings (Casey & Doherty, 2012), underscoring the importance of enhancing clinician knowledge about identifying and treating an under-researched disorder that is, in fact, quite common.

PERSISTENT COMPLEX BEREAVEMENT-RELATED DISORDER

Persistent complex bereavement-related disorder is a new diagnosis proposed for inclusion in the *DSM-5*. Based on extensive research into prolonged grief and complicated grief, APA (2013) hopes that the inclusion of this new disorder will stimulate further research into the most efficacious methods for its identification and treatment. For individuals to merit a diagnosis of persistent complex bereavement-related disorder, they must meet five criteria. Criterion A requires experiencing the death of a close relative or friend within the past year. For children, the timeframe is reduced to six months. Criterion B requires that, in the time since the death, one or more of the following symptoms is experienced often and significantly: (a) longing for the departed loved one, (b) intense feelings of sorrow, (c) preoccupation, and (d) obsessive thoughts regarding circumstances surrounding the death. In order to meet Criterion C, individuals must have experienced at least six of the following symptoms often and significantly: (a) trouble accepting the death, (b) continued feelings of shock, (c) trouble remembering the deceased positively, (d) anger over the loss, (e) self-blaming, (f) avoiding persons or places that remind the client of the death, (g) desire of joining the deceased in death, (h) trouble trusting others, (i) loneliness and detachment, (j) feelings of meaninglessness and emptiness, (k) role confusion, and (l) difficulty pursuing interests or planning for the future. The first six symptoms in Criterion C are categorized as "reactive distress to the death" while the latter six symptoms are categorized as "social/identity disruption." In order to meet Criteria D and E, the disturbance must cause substantial social, occupational, or other functional impairment, and be inconsistent with cultural norms. Clinicians should specify whether the disturbance occurs with traumatic bereavement if the individual's symptoms follow a death that occurred under traumatic circumstances.

Although much research remains to be done regarding this new disorder, some preliminary data is available. Researchers estimate that complicated grief occurs in about 10% of bereaved individuals, most commonly those with a close, identity-defining, relationship to the deceased (Zisook et al., 2010). Estimates of prolonged grief in bereaved populations also range from 9–20% (Kersting & Kroker, 2010). Those at a higher risk for developing complicated grief include females, individuals of lower income, aged 60 or above, who lost a child or a spouse, and who lost a loved one due to cancer (Kersting, Brahler, Glaesmer, & Wager, 2011).

With the exception of one groundbreaking free-access instrument which will be reviewed here, appropriate screening and assessment instruments to aid in the identification and treatment of persistent complex bereavement-related disorder remain to be developed. Future researchers should strive to develop instruments designed to differentiate this mental disorder from normal grief, mood, and anxiety disorders, and adjustment disorders.

Highlights of Free-Access Instruments Used to Identify and Monitor Outcomes

Disorders in the Trauma and Stressor-Related Disorders classification have generated an impressive amount of free-access instruments to aid in the screening, assessment, and outcome monitoring of these various disorders. Due to the overwhelmingly large number of free-access instruments in this category, only five of the very best and most commonly used instruments will be highlighted here. However, a comprehensive list at the end of the chapter will be provided for interested readers to review other trauma and stressor-related disorders instruments that might be more suited to their specific needs. The National Center for PTSD provides short reviews of many of these instruments at http://www.ptsd.va.gov/professional/pages/assessments/assessment.asp.

Stanford Acute Stress Reaction Questionnaire

The Stanford Acute Reaction Questionnaire event (SASRQ; Classen, Koopman, Hales, & Spiegel, 1998) is a self-report measure designed to assess the frequency of emotional and behavioral symptoms of acute stress disorder following a stressful event. It has been used with a wide variety of populations, including survivors of natural disasters; witnesses to, or those nearby to, acts of violence; and individuals who have received a diagnosis of cancer (Cardeña, Koopman, Classen, Waelde, & Spiegel, 2000). The SASRQ is appropriate for use with male and female adults. A version of the SASRQ modified for use with flood survivors can be found at http://stresshealthcenter.stanford.edu/research/documents/Stanford AcuteStressReactionQuestionnaire-Flood.pdf. This version can easily be adapted to any traumatic event simply by changing the wording of the initial instructions.

Administration of the SASRQ requires approximately five minutes, and can be completed in a group or individual setting. The SASRQ is composed of 30 items assessed on a six-point Likert-type scale (0 = not experienced; 1 = very rarely experienced; 2 = rarely experienced; 3 = sometimes experienced; 4 = often experienced; 5 = very often experienced) (Classen et al., 1998). One additional item at the end of the questionnaire asks the respondent to indicate the overall frequency with which these symptoms are experienced. Taken together, these items compose the five subscales of dissociation, re-experiencing of trauma, avoidance, anxiety and hyperarousal, and impairment in functioning, which closely parallel the *DSM-IV* criteria for ASD. The ASD criteria in the *DSM-5* closely mirror the criteria from *DSM-IV*, with changes in wording mainly done to mirror the language used in making PTSD diagnoses; thus, the diagnostic criteria on which the SASRQ was based are still highly appropriate and relevant. The SASRQ can either be scored dichotomously, in order to assess the presence or absence of symptoms, or using the Likert-type scale, in order to assess the severity of symptoms. Individuals are viewed as likely having ASD when they endorse at least three highly rated dissociative symptoms, as well as at least one symptom on each of the other subscales. Because the SASRQ has mainly been used as a research measure, it often serves as a reliable and efficient substitute for clinical interviews.

Scores on the SASRQ have demonstrated both reliability and validity. Test-retest reliability has been reported to be .69, and internal consistency coefficients ranged from .80 to .95 for total scores on the SASRQ (Cardeña et al., 2000; Classen et al., 1998). Construct validity is supported by the finding that individuals exposed to emergency rescues and workplace accidents obtained significantly higher scores on the SASRQ than their non-exposed peers (Cardeña, Grieger, Staab, Fullerton, & Ursano, 1997; Margiotta, Anastas, Stamm, & Everett, 1999). Additionally, SASRQ scores have been shown to increase with severity of exposure to trauma (Spiegel, Koopman, Cardeña, & Classen, 1996; Koopman, Zarcone, Mann, Freinkel, & Spiegel, 1998). In support of convergent validity, scores on the SASRQ were significantly correlated with the dissociation ($r = .68$) and anxiety ($r = .68$) subscales, as well as the total score ($r = .79$), on the Impact of Event scale (Cardeña et al., 1997). Predictive validity was evidenced by the fact that SASRQ scores obtained immediately post-flood were significantly associated with scores on the PDEQ ($r = .72$), a measure of peritraumatic dissociation, administered to flood survivors one year later (Waelde, Koopman, Rierdan, & Spiegel, 2001). Additionally, researchers have obtained a three-factor solution (dissociation, re-experiencing, and anxiety/hyperarousal), which effectively accounted for the majority of proposed subscales (Cardeña et al., 1997).

The SASRQ is advantageous mainly for measuring ASD symptomology in research settings. Given its close association with *DSM* diagnostic criteria and strong psychometrics, the SASRQ is a good choice for the efficient measurement of ASD symptoms. Additional evidence relating to the factor structure is warranted. Currently, the SASRQ should only be used with adults who have recently experienced a stressful event, and is not appropriate for use as a general population screening instrument.

Acute Stress Disorder Scale

Now the most widely used self-report measure of acute stress disorder (Edmondson, Mills, & Park, 2010), the Acute Stress Disorder Scale was originally developed as a self-report version of the Acute Stress Disorder Interview, a structured clinical interview (ASDS; Bryant, Moulds, & Guthrie, 2000). The ASDS was designed to both assess ASD and predict PTSD in adult trauma survivors, and has been translated for use in Danish (Fuglsang, Moergeli, & Schnyder, 2004), German (Helfricht et al., 2009), and Chinese (Wang, Li, Shi, Zhang, & Shen, 2010). The ASDS can be accessed as an appendix in the original article publication (Bryant et al., 2000).

The ASDS is composed of 19 items based on *DSM-IV* criteria for ASD, which align closely with *DSM-5* criteria for ASD (Bryant et al., 2000). The inventory is composed of items that reflect four subscales, including dissociation, re-experiencing, avoidance, and arousal symptoms. The respondent rates the extent to which each symptom is present on a five-point Likert-type scale ranging from 1 to 5 (1 = not at all; 2 = mildly; 3 = medium; 4 = quite a bit; 5 = very much). Total and subscale scores are obtained by summing the appropriate items. Bryant and colleagues proposed two methods of interpretation. An individual is recommended to seek additional assessment for the risk of PTSD if he or she meets either of the following criteria: (a) a score greater than, or equal to, nine on the dissociative subscale and a score greater than or equal to 28 on the re-experiencing, arousal, and avoidance subscales combined; or (b) a total raw score in excess of 56.

Psychometric evidence in support of the reliability and validity of scores on the ASDS is sound. Test-retest reliability was reported to be .94 (Bryant et al., 2000). Internal consistency coefficients for both ASDS total scores (α = .88–.96) and subscale scores (α = .62–.94) have consistently been high, with most obtained coefficients well above .70 (Bryant et al., 2000; Fuglsang et al., 2004; Helfricht et al., 2009; Wang et al., 2010). Bryant et al. reported that ASDS scores were able to identify ASD in survivors of trauma with a sensitivity of .95 and a specificity of .83.

Evidence for the convergent validity of scores on the ASDS has been provided by the numerous correlations found between ASDS total and subscale scores and scores on similar measures of post-trauma disturbance. ASDS total scores correlated strongly with ASDI total scores (*r* = .86), intrusion (*r* = .81) and avoidance (*r* = .87) subscale scores on the Impact of Events Scale, and total scores on the Beck Anxiety Inventory (*r* = .78) (Bryant et al., 2000). ASDS total scores were also moderately to highly correlated with Posttraumatic Diagnostic Scale (PDS) total scores (*r* = .72 – .88), and subscale scores on the Hospital Anxiety and Depression Scale (Anxiety: *r* = .65, Depression: *r* = .58) (Helfricht et al., 2009). Additional significant correlations were found between ASDS subscale scores and relevant subscales on these measures of psychopathology (Bryant et al., 2000; Helfricht et al., 2009).

Scores on the ASDS accurately predicted 91% of bushfire survivors who eventually developed PTSD, as well as 93% of those who did not (Bryant et al., 2000). In a later study, ASDS scores predicted only 50% of traffic accident victims who later developed high levels of PTSD symptomology (Fuglsang et al., 2004). However, although ASDS scores were only able to predict half of those who eventually developed PTSD, they were the best predictor variable in the study. Furthermore, researchers have identified a correlation of *r* = .45 between ASDS total symptom scores and PDS total symptom scores measured six months post-trauma (Helfricht et al., 2009). Although the use of an ASD diagnosis as a predictor for later PTSD has been controversial and highly criticized, it seems that the predictive validity of ASDS scores renders it the most effective method for making predictions, if one chooses to do so.

Evidence in support of construct validity is varied. Participants with ASD diagnoses scored significantly higher than both those with subclinical manifestations and those without ASD (Bryant et al., 2000; Bryant & Panasetis, 2001). However, the results of factor analysis have been inconsistent. Although Bryant and colleagues originally proposed a three- or four-factor model, subsequent researchers have found evidence of both two- (Edmondson et al., 2010) and four- (Wang et al., 2010) factor models. Each of the original four factors of dissociation, re-experiencing, avoidance, and arousal, are typically identified, but strong inter-correlations among the former three factors have allowed some to collapse these factors into a single factor to capture a better fit. Alternatively, these varied factor analysis results may reflect poor clinical understanding of the ASD construct, rather than problems with the ASDS itself.

The ASDS has marked advantages. Its basis on a structured clinical interview and *DSM-IV* criteria for ASD diagnosis highlight the strong content validity of the ASDS. As the most commonly used self-report inventory for ASD, the ASDS has been subjected to numerous psychometric evaluations and has been used with various trauma populations. This supports the applicability of the ASDS among diverse trauma populations, and also serves as a possible explanation for inconsistent factor analysis results. Given that most studies have assessed ASD with the ASDS in survivors of different traumatic events (Edmondson et al., 2010), the different factor structures obtained may indicate varied responses to stress in diverse populations, rather than an unstable general factor structure. The sole limitation of the ASDS seems to be that its use is restricted to adults.

The ASDS is a brief, psychometrically sound, self-report inventory useful for identifying trauma survivors who could benefit from a more thorough diagnostic assessment of ASD and to evaluate potential risk for PTSD. At this time, it is only appropriate for use with adults, and has mainly been used in research settings.

PTSD CHECKLIST

The PTSD Checklist (PCL) is a commonly used self-report measure of PTSD symptoms (Weathers, Litz, Herman, Huska, & Keane, 1993). The three available versions include the PTSD Checklist–Civilian (PCL-C), which is the most frequently used, the PTSD Checklist–Military (PCL-M), and the PTSD Checklist–Specific (PCL-S). The diagnostic utility of the PCL has been confirmed in various populations, including non-clinical student populations (Conybeare, Behar, Solomon, Newman, & Borkovec, 2012; Ruggiero, Del Ben, Scotti, & Rabalais, 2003), primary medical care populations (Stein, McQuaid, Pedrelli, Lenox, & McCahill, 2000; Walker, Newman, Dobie, Ciechanowski, & Katon, 2002), traffic accident and assault victims (Blanchard, Jones-Alexander, Buckley, & Forneris, 1996), individuals with cancer (Andrykowski, Cordova, Studts, & Miller, 1998; Shelby, Golden-Kreutz, & Andersen, 2005), parents of children with cancer (Manne, Du Hamel, Gallelli, Sorgen, & Redd, 1998), individuals with moderate and severe psychiatric diagnoses (Cuevas et al., 2006; Grubaugh, Elhai, Cusack, Wells, & Frueh, 2007; Mueser et al.,

2001), military veterans (Dobie et al., 2002; Williams, Monahan, & McDevitt-Murphy, 2011), firefighters (Chiu et al., 2011), and various natural disaster survivors (Hirschel & Schulenberg, 2010; Li et al., 2011). Furthermore, the PCL has been translated in both Chinese and Turkish (Kocabaşoğlu, Özdemir, Yargiç, & Geyran, 2005), and is multiculturally appropriate (Cuevas et al., 2006). The PCL was deemed suitable for use with adolescents (Wang, Dai, & Wan, 2009), adults, and the elderly (Schinka, Brown, Borenstein, & Mortimer, 2007), with or without trauma exposure. The PCL-C can be accessed at http://www.mirecc.va.gov/docs/visn6/3_PTSD_CheckList_and_Scoring.pdf.

The structure of the PCL was originally designed to reflect symptom clusters for PTSD in the *DSM-IV*. Respondents are asked to indicate the degree to which they have been bothered by each of 17 items on a five-point Likert-type scale (1 = not at all; 2 = a little bit; 3 = moderately; 4 = quite a bit; 5 = extremely). All items are summed to obtain a total score, which is the most common scoring method. Various cut-off scores have been proposed for different populations, but it is most common to use a cut-point of 44 in civilian populations and 50 in military populations (McDonald & Calhoun, 2010). The symptom cluster scoring method requires the scorer to treat any responses ranging from three to five (moderately or above) as symptomatic. Then, in order for a respondent to screen positively, he must indicate at least one Criterion B item (items 1–5), at least three Criterion C items (items 6–12), and at least two Criterion D items (items 13–17). Respondents who exceed either of these two scoring thresholds screen positively for PTSD. Because a self-report inventory is insufficient for diagnosis of PTSD, the PCL is not appropriate for use as a diagnostic tool. Instead, individuals who screen positively on the PCL are at heightened risk of PTSD due to high symptomology, and should seek further diagnostic assessment via a structured clinical interview.

Evidence in support of the reliability and validity of scores on the various versions of the PCL is abundant (Wilkins, Lang, & Norman, 2011). Weathers et al. (1993) originally reported a test-retest reliability coefficient of .96 in traffic accident and sexual assault survivors. Test-retest reliability coefficients in nonclinical student populations were similarly high after a short passage of time (r = .92 for immediate retest; r = .88 for one week interval), but dropped considerably after two weeks

($r = .66–.68$) (Conybeare et al., 2012; Ruggiero et al., 2003). The internal consistency of PCL scores is exceptionally high, with α coefficients above .92 for the total score and above .80 for most symptom cluster scores (Blanchard et al., 1996; Conybeare et al., 2012; Cuevas et al., 2006; Mueser et al., 2001; Ruggiero et al., 2003; Weathers et al.). Sensitivity and specificity values vary across settings and populations (McDonald & Calhoun, 2010). With cut-points specific to maximizing these values in different populations ranging from 30 to 60, researchers have obtained optimal sensitivities ranging from .32–1.00 and specificities ranging from .86–.99 (Andrykowski et al., 1998; Blanchard et al., 1996; Chiu et al., 2011; Dobie et al., 2002; Grubaugh et al., 2007; Manne et al., 1998; McDonald & Calhoun, 2010; Stein et al., 2000; Walker et al., 2002). Higher cut-points seem appropriate in populations with more severe psychiatric illness (Grubaugh et al., 2007), likely because a higher cut-point is necessary to distinguish PTSD from a myriad of overlapping symptoms from comorbid conditions. Lower cut-scores enhance sensitivity outside acute trauma settings (Walker et al., 2002), and Stein et al. (2000) advocated strongly for lowered screening thresholds in order to accurately identify all cases of PTSD. However, although cut-points are expected to vary by population in order to maximize accuracy in each (Dobie et al., 2002), the lack of an agreed upon cut-off score is problematic (Ruggiero et al., 2003). Ruggiero et al. recommend a cut-off score of 44 to maximize utility in the majority of populations, but McDonald and Calhoun (2010) warn that strict reliance on one proposed cut-off score over another could lead to flawed results. Thus, clinicians and researchers who wish to use the PCL are advised to determine the most appropriate published cut-points for their specific population.

Although the diagnostic utility of the PCL is variable, evidence for the convergent and discriminant validity of the PCL is more favorable. Moderate to high correlations have been documented among PCL total and subscale scores with both self-report measures of PTSD symptomology, such as the Impact of Event Scale ($r = .77$; Ruggiero et al., 2003), the Trauma Symptoms Checklist ($r = .60$; Conybeare et al., 2012), and the Mississippi Scale for PTSD—Civilian version ($r = .82$; Ruggiero et al., 2003), and clinician interviews, such as the gold standard Clinician-Administered PTSD Scale ($r = .92$; Blanchard et al., 1996; Grubaugh et al., 2007; Mueser et al., 2001). Correlations between the PCL and the IES were significantly higher than PCL correlations with several other measures of depression and various domains of psychopathology (Ruggiero et al., 2003). Furthermore, the PCL has been shown to be superior to other similar measures in discriminating between symptoms of trauma and symptoms of anxiety, obsessive-compulsive disorder, and depression (Conybeare et al., 2012).

Numerous researchers have examined the factor structure of the PCL. Although researchers have found one-, two-, three-, and four-factor solutions (Conybeare et al., 2012; Cuevas et al., 2006; Palmieri, Weathers, Difede, & King, 2007; Schinka et al., 2007; Shelby et al., 2005; Wang et al., 2009), the four-factor model is by far the most commonly found factor structure of the PCL (Wilkins et al., 2011). This initially seems troubling, given that the item construction of the PCL was predicated on the underlying PTSD structure of three factors: re-experiencing, avoidance, and arousal. However, the three PTSD symptom clusters identified in the *DSM-IV* are expanded to four symptom clusters in the *DSM-5* (APA, 2013). Thus, the four-factor structure typically identified in the PCL actually reflects the recently updated underlying structure of the PTSD construct, which now includes negative changes in cognitions and mood (Williams et al., 2011). Gauci and MacDonald (2012) confirmed the suitability of a four-factor model for the PCL in a large, heterogeneous population with exposure to various different types of trauma. Therefore, the existing structure of the PCL aligns well with the new *DSM-5* criteria for PTSD, rendering it the instrument of choice for appropriately assessing PTSD consistent with the new criteria.

The advantages of the PCL are manifold, but it has some disadvantages as well. The various versions of the PCL allow the researcher or clinician to determine which version provides the best fit to meet desired goals in a given population. The PCL-C is able to tap multiple trauma experiences, while the PCL-S is advantageous in confirming that at least one specific trauma meets PTSD criteria for a traumatic experience (McDonald & Calhoun, 2010). The PCL-M is useful for traumatic experiences encountered while in the military, but may miss non-military traumas in military members.

Although it was developed in the 1990s, the PCL already reflects the underlying structure of PTSD symptom clusters outlined in the *DSM-5*, even though it does not assess every criterion required for diagnosis of

PTSD. The PCL is thus ideally suited to continue to accurately screen for PTSD symptomology. However, researchers and clinicians are cautioned that using the symptom cluster scoring method would likely no longer prove to be a viable option unless scoring guidelines were reworked to reflect the four symptom-clusters of the *DSM-5*. In addition, given that it is still unclear what the minimum score should be to constitute meeting PTSD criteria (Ruggiero et al., 2003), researchers and clinicians are charged with the task of choosing an appropriate cut-score with the extant information in the literature as a guide, but not an answer.

Various researchers have found the PCL to have greater diagnostic utility than other, shorter, screening tests, such as the SPAN and the PC-PTSD (McDonald & Calhoun, 2010). Some researchers have even attempted to develop shortened versions of the PCL, and have offered preliminary evidence for the psychometric adequacy of two- and six-item versions (Lang & Stein, 2005). However, other researchers failed to find adequate psychometric support for these abbreviated versions (Hirschel & Schulenberg, 2010). At this time, the full 17-item version of the PCL is backed by copious evidence of strong psychometrics, and offers impressive brevity as well. Until additional evidence substantiates the utility of abbreviated versions, the full PCL remains the PTSD self-report inventory of choice.

The PCL is useful both as a screening device to assess the possible presence of PTSD and as a measure for tracking change in symptoms over time (McDonald & Calhoun, 2010). Backed by an abundance of psychometric support, the PCL is the best available self-report screening instrument for assessing PTSD symptoms, and it is most useful if it is paired with a follow-up diagnostic interview. Researchers and clinicians should strive to educate themselves about the most applicable cut-off scores for their specific populations.

PTSD SYMPTOM SCALE

The PTSD Symptom Scale is a brief screening inventory designed to assess the frequency and severity of PTSD symptoms (PSS; Foa, Riggs, Dancu, & Rothbaum, 1993). Both the interview (PSS-I) and self-report (PSS-SR) versions have been used with individuals with diverse trauma histories, including assault victims (Foa et al., 1993), crime victims

(Wohlfarth, van den Brink, Winkel, & ter Smitten, 2003), traffic accident survivors (Coffey, Gudmundsdottir, Beck, Palyo, & Miller, 2006), earthquake survivors (Foa, Johnson, Feeny, & Treadwell, 2001), military veterans (Nacasch et al., 2007), parents of children with high-risk medical diagnoses (Landolt, Boehler, Schwager, Schallberger, & Nuessli, 1998), individuals recovering from first-episode psychosis (Sin, Abdin, & Lee, 2012), and individuals with comorbid substance abuse (Coffey, Dansky, Falsetti, Saladin, & Brady, 1998; Powers, Gillihan, Rosenfield, Jerud, & Foa, 2012). A revised version, the MPSS-SR, was modified to include severity ratings (Falsetti, Resnick, Resick, & Kilpatrick, 1993). Available in multiple languages, the PSS-I and the PSS-SR are both intended for use with adults (Foa et al., 1993), while the Child PTSD Symptom Scale (CPSS) is appropriate for use with children and adolescents aged 8 to 18 (Foa et al., 2001). The PSS-SR is available at http://depts.washington.edu/hcsats/PDF/TF-%20CBT/pages/1%20Assessment/Standardized%20Measures/PSS-Adult.pdf. The other versions of the PSS can be accessed by contacting the principal authors of the respective versions and requesting a copy.

The PSS only requires approximately 10 to 15 minutes for completion. The PSS is composed of 17 items which are directly aligned with the *DSM-IV* criteria for PTSD (Foa et al., 1993); thus, items correspond to the three symptom clusters of re-experiencing, avoidance, and arousal. Respondents or interviewers rate items designed to assess symptom frequency over the past two weeks according to a four-point Likert-type scale (0 = not at all; 1 = once a week/a little bit/once in a while; 2 = two to four times per week/somewhat/half the time; 3 = five or more times per week/very much/almost always). Symptoms scored as a one or higher are considered present. Diagnosis of PTSD is confirmed if respondents endorse at least one re-experiencing symptom, at least three avoidance symptoms, and at least two arousal symptoms. A total score, calculated by summing all items, can also be calculated as an index of symptom severity. Researchers who have used the PSS for screening have recommended various total score cut-offs. Cut-scores of 14 are most typical (Coffey et al., 2006; Sin et al., 2012), while lower cut-scores of 11 are more appropriate for children (Foa et al., 2001), and higher cut-scores of 28 are more appropriate for adults with comorbid diagnoses (Coffey et al., 1998).

Scores on the PSS have robust evidence of both reliability and validity. They are temporally stable, with test-retest reliability coefficients ranging from .80 to .84 (Foa et al., 2001; Powers et al., 2012). Interrater reliability is excellent, with both total and subscale coefficients in the .90s (Foa & Tolin, 2000). Good to excellent internal consistency coefficients have also been reported for both total scores (α = .89–.97) and subscale scores (α = .65–.95) (Coffey et al., 1998; Foa & Tolin, 2000; Foa et al., 2001; Powers et al., 2012). Foa and Tolin (2012) found the internal consistency of the PSS-I, along with its other psychometric properties, to be on par with the excellent psychometric properties of the CAPS, the gold standard in PTSD diagnosis.

Furthermore, the diagnostic utility of scores on the PSS is quite good. Sensitivity has ranged from .80 to .91, while specificity has been lower, ranging from .62 to .90 (Coffey et al., 1998; Coffey et al., 2006; Foa & Tolin, 2012; Powers et al., 2012; Sin et al., 2012; Wohlfarth et al., 2003). In a study by Foa et al. (2001), the sensitivity and specificity of scores on the CPSS were .95 and .96, respectively. However, Engelhard, Arntz, and van den Hout (2007) found the markedly lower specificity of .43 on the PSS, due to the fact that individuals with an anxiety disorder often falsely screened positive.

Scores on the PSS demonstrate excellent concurrent, convergent, and divergent validity. Good concurrent validity was originally reported with SCID diagnoses (Falsetti et al., 1993; Foa et al., 1993), and more recent research confirmed concurrent validity with high correlations with the SCID (r = .73, kappa = .75), the CAPS (r = .87) (Foa & Tolin, 2000; Powers et al., 2012). Convergent validity has been evidenced by correlations between PSS total scores and scores on similar measures of symptoms in response to trauma, including the SCL-90-R PTSD Scale (r = .79), the IES (r = .66), and the PDS (r = .78) (Coffey et al., 1998; Powers et al.). Correlations among relevant subscales have been similarly high. Researchers also obtained a .80 correlation between scores on the CPSS and the Child Posttraumatic Stress Disorder Reaction Index (CPTSD-RI) (Foa et al., 2001). Divergent validity is evidenced by the lower correlations obtained among PSS scores and measures of depression and anxiety (Foa et al., 2001).

There is a dearth of research regarding the factor structure of the PSS. This is surprising given that both the PSS and the PCL are based off of the same *DSM-IV* PTSD criteria, yet the factor structure of the PSS remains largely uninvestigated, while the factor structure of the PCL has been examined profusely. At this point, most researchers have failed to support the latent three-factor structure proposed by the *DSM-IV*, and have instead suggested that a four-factor model composed of intrusion, avoidance, numbing, and hyper-arousal factors fits better (Naifeh, Elhai, Kashdan, & Grubaugh, 2008). However, these four factors do not align as well with the *DSM-5* criteria as those of the PCL.

There are both pros and cons inherent in the use of the PSS. The fact that the PSS is able to index both symptom frequency and severity is impressive. The multiple versions available allow researchers and clinicians the capacity to administer either individual interviews or self-report versions in an individual or group setting, depending on which version is most appropriate to their setting and purpose. The inclusion of a version adapted for use with children and adolescents renders the PSS extremely useful. The children's version even includes additional dichotomous questions designed to assess functional impairment, bringing the CPSS even closer to the *DSM* diagnostic criteria for PTSD (Foa et al., 2001). Given the abundant evidence documenting the strong psychometrics of the PSS, as well as the finding that the PSS-I performed equally well to the CAPS, but in a much shorter assessment time (Foa & Tolin, 2000), the PSS is clearly an excellent alternative to the CAPS when professionals wish to save time and money. Some have even suggested that individual items on the PSS may be just as accurate in predicting PTSD as the full scale (Wohlfarth et al., 2003), but additional psychometric evaluation is needed. However, given the recent changes in diagnostic criteria for PTSD in the *DSM-5* and the lack of definitive evidence in support of the factor structure of the PSS, future researchers need to validate the latent structure of the PSS with *DSM-5* criteria to ensure proper alignment. Although the PSS is effective at distinguishing individuals with PTSD from non-PTSD controls, professionals are cautioned to be aware of the low specificity of the PSS in distinguishing PTSD from other psychopathology (Engelhard et al., 2007).

In conclusion, the various versions of the PSS provide excellent options for assessing PTSD symptom frequency and severity in a wide variety of populations in both research and clinical settings. The PSS-I has demonstrated equality with the gold standard diagnostic interview, the CAPS (Foa & Tolin, 2000), and can also be used as an outcome measure to assess change post-treatment (Nacasch et al., 2011). Although potential users are cautioned that self-report inventories are not appropriate as a sole basis for diagnosis, the interview version renders the PSS useful for both screening and diagnosis (Powers et al., 2012). Thus, professionals wishing to assign diagnoses must either choose the interview version or follow the self-report version with a clinician-administered interview. Additional evidence of the factor structure and most appropriate cut-scores would serve to further improve the robust psychometric properties of the PSS.

Inventory of Complicated Grief

Created by one of the leading researchers in the newly emerging field of complicated grief, the Inventory of Complicated Grief (ICG) was developed to assess the symptoms of complicated grief in order to differentiate between normal and complicated grievers (Prigerson et al., 1995). Prigerson et al. defined complicated grief symptoms as those that differ from depression- and anxiety-related bereavement and predict enduring functional impairments. Thus, converse to other extant grief assessment measures, the ICG was designed to measure only maladaptive, not normative, symptoms of grief, in order to serve as a predictive screening and/or diagnostic instrument. Numerous researchers have adapted the ICG for their specific purposes, resulting in modified versions which are appropriate for use with children and adolescents aged 7 to 18 years (Melhem, Moritz, Walker, Shear, & Brent, 2007), adults with intellectual disabilities (Guerin et al., 2009), and adults who are grieving the loss of a companion pet (King & Werner, 2012). The original ICG and the ICG-Revised (Prigerson & Jacobs, 2001) have been used with adults who have suffered the loss of a spouse (Prigerson et al., 1995) or a child (Dyregrov, Mortensen, & Dyregrov, 2003), as well as with both general population and psychiatric clinic samples of individuals who have experienced a significant loss due to both violent and natural causes of death (Boelen & van den Bout, 2007; Mitchell, Kim, Prigerson, & Mortimer-Stephens, 2004; Prigerson et al., 2002). The ICG and ICG-R are thus appropriate for use among various populations of grieving adults and can be accessed as an appendix in the original journal article publication.

The ICG is composed of 19 items which assess emotional, cognitive, and behavioral symptoms of complicated grief on a five-point Likert-type scale (0 = never; 1 = rarely; 2 = sometimes; 3 = often; 4 = always) (Prigerson et al., 1995). The items accommodate the responses of elderly individuals who may have diminished memory capacity by phrasing items to assess the current time frame, as opposed to an earlier, extended, time period. ICG items are summed to obtain a total score. Prigerson et al. classified individuals who met or exceeded the diagnostic threshold score of 25 as cases of complicated grief. When using the ICG-R, administrators should classify individuals as complicated grievers if they meet the following criteria: (a) at least three of four separation distress (Criterion A2) symptoms are endorsed at least "frequently," (b) at least four of eight traumatic distress (Criterion B) symptoms are endorsed at least "frequently," and (c) functional impairment (Criterion D) is endorsed at least "sometimes" (Boelen & van den Bout, 2007).

Initial evidence of the reliability and validity of scores on the ICG and the ICG-R is promising. The test-retest reliability coefficient was .80 after a six-month interval (Prigerson et al., 1995), and internal consistency coefficients have continually exceeded .92 (King & Werner, 2012; Melhem et al., 2007; Prigerson et al., 1995; Prigerson et al., 2002). Sensitivities ranging from .73 to .93 and specificities ranging from .93 to .99 showcase the diagnostic utility of scores on the ICG and the ICG-R (Boelen & van den Bout, 2007; Prigerson et al., 1999). Scores on the ICG were significantly correlated with scores on various measures of general grief, depression, and anxiety symptoms, including the Texas Revised Inventory of Grief (r = .87), the Beck Depression Inventory (r = .67), and the Grief Measurement Scale (r = .70), providing evidence of convergent validity (Prigerson et al., 1995). Scores on the ICG-R were also significantly correlated with symptoms of depression, anxiety, hopelessness, PTSD, suicidal ideation, and both self-ratings and clinical ratings of functional impairment (Melhem et al., 2007). Furthermore, individuals with scores in excess of the cut-point scored significantly lower on quality of life and overall mental health measures and significantly higher on depressive severity measures, providing support for construct validity (Ott, 2003; Prigerson et al., 1995). In addition, factor analysis has generally supported the one-factor structure on which the ICG was based (Boelen & Hoijtink, 2009; Prigerson et al., 1995), with few exceptions (Melhem et al., 2007).

The underlying factor structure of the ICG and, most importantly, the construct of complicated grief, should be given further attention in the future.

The ICG and ICG-R are advantageous for many reasons. The criteria for traumatic grief on which these instruments are based closely mirror the proposed *DSM-5* criteria for persistent complex bereavement disorder (APA, 2013; Prigerson et al., 1999). Future evidence of factor structure will likely confirm that the construct of complicated grief is appropriately reflected in the item construction of the ICG and the ICG-R. Ideally, a better understanding of the construct of complicated grief will also help researchers to choose a single clear method for ICG score interpretation, since past recommendations have yet to reach a clear consensus (Boelen & van den Bout, 2007; Ott, 2003; Prigerson et al., 1995; Prigerson et al., 2002). Moreover, items on these instruments function well across genders and individuals bereaving a variety of types of losses (Boelen & Hoijtink, 2009). In addition to its utility in screening and diagnosis, the ICG has also been used to obtain prevalence estimates (Prigerson et al., 2002) and as an outcome evaluation measure post-treatment (Dyregrov et al., 2003). Given past evidence that the ICG performs better than the TRIG when differentiating people with various levels of impairment (Prigerson et al., 1995), the ICG seems to be the clear choice for assessing complicated grief.

The ICG and its various alternate versions are thus highly recommended for use in the screening and diagnostic assessment of complicated grief in bereaved individuals. Because persistent complex grief disorder is a new disorder in the *DSM-5*, the ICG will be useful in calculating prevalence estimates, screening bereaved individuals, and both planning and assessing treatment options. Considering the substantial overlap between diagnostic criteria and the symptoms outlined in the ICG, the ICG is well suited to the assessment of complicated grief symptoms. However, clinicians are cautioned that self-report inventories should always be followed with a clinical interview for diagnosis. Given that a clinical interview does not yet exist for the assessment of persistent complex bereavement disorder, clinicians are advised to supplement the results of the ICG with as much information as possible.

Additional Free-Access Instruments Which May Be Suitable for Diverse Needs

Trauma and stressor-related disorders have spawned an incredible amount of clinical interest and an impressive number of free-access instruments, surely the most of any of the diagnostic categories in this book. Due to the large number of free-access instruments available, a list is provided here of various instruments which may be more appropriate for research or clinical applications with specific trauma populations (e.g., Combat Exposure Scale) or to confirm the existence of traumatic events prior to assessing for symptoms (e.g., Life Events Checklist). Many of these instruments are likely extremely useful, but were not selected for review due to an unacceptably small amount of psychometric data and minimal usage in the literature. It should be emphasized that the instruments reviewed above represent the best available instruments for assessing a wide variety of populations for specific symptoms, but researchers may alternatively wish to use any of the following instruments, all of which can be found using any search engine or in the professional literature. Short reviews of many of these instruments are provided at http://www.ptsd.va.gov/professional/pages/assessments/assessment.asp.

- Accident Fear Questionnaire
- Acute Stress Checklist for Children (ASC-Kids)
- Afghan Symptom Checklist
- Brief Grief Questionnaire
- Children's Impact of Traumatic Events Scale—Revised
- Combat Exposure Scale
- Grief Evaluation Measure
- Harvard Trauma Questionnaire
- Impact of Event Scale
- Life Events Checklist
- Primary Care—PTSD Screen (PC-PTSD)
- Posttraumatic Cognitions Inventory
- PTSD-8
- Structured Clinical Interview for Trauma and Loss Spectrum (SCI-TALS)
- Stressful Life Events Screening Questionnaire

- Texas Revised Inventory of Grief (TRIG)
- Traumatic Event Screening Inventory
- Trauma History Questionnaire
- Trauma History Screen

References

Aalto, M., Alho, H., Halme, J., & Seppä, K. (2011). The Alcohol Use Disorders Identification Test (AUDIT) and its derivatives in screening for heavy drinking among the elderly. *International Journal of Geriatric Psychiatry, 26,* 881–885. doi: 10.1002/gps.2498

Achenbach, T. M., & Rescorla, L. A. (2001). *Manual for the Achenbach System of Empirically Based Assessment (ASEBA)*. Burlington, VT: ASEBA.

Adler, L. A., Spencer, T., Faraone, S. V., Kessler, R. C., Howes, M. J., Biederman, J., & Secnik, K. (2006). Validity of pilot Adult AD/HD Self-Report Scale (ASRS) to rate adult AD/HD symptoms. *Annals of Clinical Psychiatry, 18*(3), 145–148. doi: 10.1080/10401230600801077

Ali, R., Awwad, E., Babor, T., Bradley, F., Butau, T., Farrell, M., ...Vendetti, J. (2002). The Alcohol, Smoking, and Substance Involvement Screening Test (ASSIST): Development, reliability, and feasibility. *Addiction, 97,* 1183–1194.

Allison, C., Auyeung, B., & Baron-Cohen, S. (2012). Toward brief "red flags" for autism screening: The short Autism Spectrum Quotient and the short Quantitative Checklist in 1,000 cases and 3,000 controls. *Journal of the American Academy of Child & Adolescent Psychiatry, 51,* 202–212. doi: 10.1016/j.jaac.2011.11.003

Allison, D. B., Kalinsky, L. B., & Gorman, B. S. (1992). A comparison of the psychometric properties of three measures of dietary restraint. *Psychological Assessment, 4,* 391–398.

Ambrosini, P. J. (2000). Historical development and present status of the Schedule for Affective Disorders and Schizophrenia for school-age children (K-SADS). *Journal of the American Academy of Child & Adolescent Psychiatry, 39,* 49–58.

American Psychiatric Association. (1980). *Diagnostic and statistical manual of mental disorders* (3rd ed.). Washington, DC: Author.

American Psychiatric Association. (1994). *Diagnostic and statistical manual of mental disorders* (4th ed.). Washington, DC: Author.

American Psychiatric Association. (2013). *Diagnostic and statistical manual of mental disorders* (5th ed.). Washington, DC: Author.

Anastasi, A., & Urbina, S. (1997). *Psychological testing.* Upper Saddle River, NJ: Prentice Hall.

Andrykowski, M. A., Cordova, M. J., Studts, J. L., & Miller, T. W. (1998). Posttraumatic stress disorder after treatment for breast cancer: Prevalence of diagnosis and use of the PTSD Checklist–Civilian version (PCL-C) as a screening instrument. *Journal of Consulting and Clinical Psychology, 66*, 586–590.

Antony, M. M., Coons, M. J., McCabe, R. E., Ashbaugh, A., & Swinson, R. P. (2006). Psychometric properties of the Social Phobia Inventory: Further evaluation. *Behaviour Research and Therapy, 44*, 1177–1185.

Austin, E. J. (2004). Personality correlates of the broader autism phenotype as assessed by the Autism Spectrum Quotient (AQ). *Personality and Individual Differences, 38*, 451–460. doi: 10.1016/j.paid.2004.04.022

Auyeung, B., Baron-Cohen, S., Wheelwright, S., & Allison, C. (2008). The Autism Spectrum Quotient–Children's version (AQ-Child). *Journal of Autism and Developmental Disorders, 38*, 1230–1240. doi: 10.1007/s10803-007-0504-z

Bagby, R. M., Ryder, A. G., Schuller, D. R., & Marshall, M. B. (2004). The Hamilton Depression Rating Scale: Has the gold standard become a lead weight? *American Journal of Psychiatry, 161*, 2163–2177. doi: 10.1176/appi.ajp.161.12.2163

Baron-Cohen, S., Hoekstra, R. A., Knickmeyer, R., & Wheelwright, S. (2006). The Autism-Spectrum Quotient (AQ)–Adolescent version. *Journal of Autism & Developmental Disorders, 36*, 343–350. doi: 10.1007/s10803-006-0073-6

Baron-Cohen, S., Lombardo, M. V., Auyeung, B., Ashwin, E., Chakrabarti, B., & Knickmeyer, R. (2011). Why are autism spectrum conditions more prevalent in males? *PLOS Biology, 9*, 1–10.

Baron-Cohen, S., Wheelwright, S., Skinner, R., Martin, J., & Clubley, E. (2001). The Autism-Spectrum Quotient (AQ): Evidence from Asperger syndrome/high-functioning autism, males and females, scientists and mathematicians. *Journal of Autism and Developmental Disorders, 31*, 5–17.

Barrett, R., & Fritz, G. K. (2010). DSM-5 and autism. *The Brown University Child & Adolescent Behavior Letter, 26*, 8.

Bauer, S., Winn, S., Schmidt, U., & Kordy, H. (2005). Construction, scoring and validation of the short evaluation of eating disorders (seed). *European Eating Disorders Review, 13*, 191–200. doi: 10.1002/erv.637

Beck, A. T., & Steer, R. A. (1991). Relationship between the Beck Anxiety Inventory and the Hamilton Anxiety Rating Scale with anxious outpatients. *Journal of Anxiety Disorders, 5*, 213–223.

Beck, J. G., & Coffey, S. F. (2007). Assessment and treatment of posttraumatic stress disorder after a motor vehicle collision: Empirical findings and clinical observations. *Professional Psychology: Research and Practice, 38*, 629–639. doi: 10.1037/0735-7028.38.6.629

Benvenuti, P., Ferrara, M., Niccolai, C., Valoriani, V., & Cox, J. L. (1999). The Edinburgh Postnatal Depression Scale: Validation for an Italian sample. *Journal of Affective Disorders, 53*, 137–141.

Berner, M. M., Kriston, L., Bentele, M., & Harter, M. (2007). The Alcohol Use Disorders Identification Test for detecting at-risk drinking: A systematic review and meta-analysis. *Journal of Studies on Alcohol and Drugs, 68*, 461–473.

Bernos-Hernandez, M. N., Rodriguez-Ruiz, S., Perez, M., Gleaves, D. H., Maysonet, M., & Cepeda-Benito, A. (2007). Cross-cultural assessment of eating disorders: Psychometric properties of a Spanish version of the bulimia test-revised. *European Eating Disorders Review, 15*, 418–424. doi: 10.1002/erv.791

Birmaher, B., Ehmann, M., Axelson, D. A., Goldstein, B. I., Monk, K., Kalas, C., ... Brent, D. A. (2009). Schedule for Affective Disorders and Schizophrenia for School-Age Children (K-SADS-PL) for the assessment of preschool children - A preliminary psychometric study. *Journal of Psychiatric Research, 43*, 680–686.

Bizzarri, J. V., Benedetti, A., Rucci, P., Scarpellini, P., Dilani, F., Milanti, M., Massei, G. J., ... Cassano, G. B. (2009). Comorbidity with anxiety and substance use disorders in patients with schizophrenia. *Giornale Italiano di Psicopatologia, 15*, 120–125.

Blanchard, E. B., Jones-Alexander, J., Buckley, T. C., & Forneris, C. A. (1996). Psychometric properties of the PTSD Checklist (PCL). *Behavior Research and Therapy, 34*, 669–673. doi: 10.1016/0005-7967(96)00033-2

Bloom, L. (1998). Review of the Eating Inventory. In J. C. Impara & B. S. Plake (Eds.), *The thirteenth mental measurements yearbook*. Retrieved from http://www.buros.unl.edu

Boelen, P. A., & Hoijtink, H. (2009). An item response theory analysis of a measure of complicated grief. *Death Studies, 33*, 101–129. doi: 10.1080/07481180802602758

Boelen, P. A., & van den Bout, J. (2007). Examination of proposed criteria for complicated grief in people confronted with violent or non-violent loss. *Death Studies, 31*, 155–164. doi: 10.1080/07481180601100541

Boschloo, L, Vogelzangs, N., Smit, J. H., van den Brink, W., Veltman, D. J., Beekman, A. T. F., & Penninx, B. W. (2010). The performance of the Alcohol Use Disorder Identification Test (AUDIT) in detecting alcohol abuse and dependence in a population of depressed or anxious persons. *Journal of Affective Disorders, 126*, 441–446. doi: 10.1016/j.jad.2010.04.019

Bowles, S. V., Bernard, R. S., Epperly, T., Woodward, S., Ginzburg, K., Folen, R., ... Koopman, C. (2006). Traumatic stress disorders following first-trimester spontaneous abortion: A pilot study of patient characteristics associated with these disorders. *The Journal of Family Practice, 55*, 969–973.

Braaten, K., Briegleb, C., Hauke, S., Niamkey, N., & Chang, G. (2008). Screening pregnant young adults for alcohol and drug use: A pilot study. *Journal of Addiction Medicine, 2*, 74–78. doi: 10.1097/ADM.0b013e31815e4f7b

Brelsford, T. N., Hummel, R. M., & Barrios, B. A. (1992). The Bulimia Test-Revised: A psychometric investigation. *Psychological Assessment, 4*, 399–401.

Brewin, C. R., Andrews, B., Rose, S., & Kirk, M. (1999). Acute stress disorder and posttraumatic stress disorder in victims of violent crime. *The American Journal of Psychiatry, 156*, 360–366.

Brown, C., Schulberg, H. C., & Madonia, M. J. (1995). Assessing depression in primary care practice with the Beck Depression Inventory and the Hamilton Rating Scale for Depression. *Psychological Assessment, 7*, 59–65.

Brugha, T. S., McManus, S., Smith, J., Scott, F. J., Meltzer, H., Purdon, S., ... Bankart, J. (2012). Validating two survey methods for identifying cases of autism spectrum disorder among adults in the community. *Psychological Medicine: A Journal of Research in Psychiatry and the Allied Sciences, 42*, 647–656. doi: 10.1017/S0033291711001292

Bruss, G. S., Gruenberg, A. M., Goldstein, R. D., & Barber, J. P. (1994). Hamilton Anxiety Rating Scale interview guide: Joint interview and test-retest methods for interrater reliability. *Psychiatry Research, 53*, 191–202.

Bryant, R. A. (2011). Acute stress disorder as a predictor of posttraumatic stress disorder: A systematic review. *Journal of Clinical Psychiatry, 72*, 233–239. doi: 10.4088/JCP.09r05072blu

Bryant, R. A., Creamer, M., O'Donnell, M., Silove, D., & McFarlane, A. C. (2012). The capacity of acute stress disorder to predict posttraumatic psychiatric disorders. *Journal of Psychiatric Research, 46*, 168–173. doi: 10.1016/j.jpsychires.2011.10.007

Bryant, R. A., Moulds, M. L., & Guthrie, R. M. (2000). Acute Stress Disorder Scale: A self-report measure of acute stress disorder. *Psychological Assessment, 12*, 61–68. doi: 10.1037/1040-3590.12.1.61

Bryant, R. A., & Panasetis, P. (2001). Panic symptoms during trauma and acute stress disorder. *Behaviour Research and Therapy, 39*, 961–966. doi: 10.1016/S0005-7967(00)00086-3

Bryant, R. A., Salmon, K., Sinclair, E., & Davidson, P. (2007). The relationship between acute stress disorder and posttraumatic stress disorder in injured children. *Journal of Traumatic Stress, 20*, 1075–1079. doi: 10.1002/jts.20282

Bussing, R., Fernandez, M., Harwood, M., Hou, W., Garvan, C. W., Eyberg, S. M., & Swanson, J. M. (2008). Parent and teacher SNAP-IV ratings of Attention Deficit Hyperactivity Disorder symptoms: Psychometric properties and normative ratings from a school district sample. *Assessment, 15*, 317–328.

Byun, S., Ruffini, C., Mills, J. E., Douglas, A. C., Niang, M., Stepchenkova, S., ... Blanton, M. (2009). Internet addiction: Metasynthesis of 1996–2006 quantitative research. *CyberPsychology & Behavior, 12*, 203–207. doi: 10.1089/cpb.2008.0102

Cabizuca, M., Marques-Portella, C., Mendlowicz, M. V., Coutinho, E. S. F., & Figueira, I. (2009). Posttraumatic stress disorder in parents of children with chronic illnesses: A meta-analysis. *Health Psychology, 28*, 379–388. doi: 10.1037/a0014512

Caci, H. M., Bouchez, J., & Bayle, F. J. (2010). An aid for diagnosing attention-deficit/hyperactivity disorder at adulthood: Psychometric properties of the French versions of two Wender Utah Rating Scales (WURS-25 and WURS-K). *Comprehensive Psychiatry, 51*(3), 325–331.

Campbell, J. M. (2005). Diagnostic assessment of Asperger's disorder: A review of five third-party rating scales. *Journal of Autism & Developmental Disorders, 35*, 25–35. doi: 10.1007/s10803-004-1028-4

Campbell-Sills, L., Norman, S. B., Craske, M. G., Sullivan, G., Lang, A. J., Chavira, D. A., ... Stein, M. B. (2009). Validation of a brief measure of anxiety-related severity and impairment: The Overall Anxiety Severity and Impairment Scale (OASIS). *Journal of Affective Disorders, 112*, 92–101. doi: 10.1016/j.jad.2008.03.014

Campo-Arias, A., Díaz-Martínez, L. A., Rueda-Jaimes, G. E., del Pilar Cadena, L., & Hernández, N. L. (2006). Validation of Zung's Self-Rating Depression Scale among the Colombian general population. *Social Behavior and Personality, 34*, 87–94.

Canal-Bedia, R., García-Primo, P., Martín-Cilleros, M. V., Santos-Borbujo, J., Guisuraga-Fernández, Z., Herráez-García, L., ... Posada-de la Paz, M. (2011). Modified Checklist for Autism in Toddlers: Cross-cultural adaptation and validation in Spain. *Journal of Autism and Developmental Disorders, 41*, 1342–1351. doi: 10.1007/s10803-010-1163-z

Canals, J., Carbajo, G., & Fernandez-Ballart, J. (2002). Discriminant validity of the Eating Attitudes Test according to American Psychiatric Association and the World Health Organization criteria of eating disorders. *Psychological Reports, 91*, 1052–1056.

Cappelleri, J. C., Bushmakin, A. G., Gerber, R. A., Leidy, N. K., Sexton, C. C., Lowe, M. R., & Karlsson, J. (2009). Psychometric analysis of the Three-Factor Eating Questionnaire-R21: Results from a large diverse sample of obese and non-obese participants. *International Journal of Obesity, 33*, 611–620.

Cardeña, E., Koopman, C., Classen, C., Waelde, L. C., & Spiegel, D. (2000). Psychometric properties of the Stanford Acute Stress Reaction Questionnaire (SASRQ): A valid and reliable measure of acute stress. *Journal of Traumatic Stress, 13*, 719–734.

Cardeña, E., Grieger, T., Staab, J., Fullerton, C., & Ursano, R. (1997). Memory disturbances in the acute aftermath of disasters. In J. D. Read, & D. S. Lindsay (Eds.), *Recollections of trauma* (p. 568). New York, NY: Plenum.

Carlson, M., Wilcox, R., Chou, C., Chang, M., Yang, F., Blanchard, J., ... Clark, F. (2011). Psychometric properties of reverse-scored items on the CES-D in a sample of ethnically diverse older adults. *Psychological Assessment, 23*, 558–562. doi: 10.1037/a0022484

Carmody, T. J., Rush, A. J., Bernstein, I., Warden, D., Brannan, S., Burnham, D., Woo, A., & Trivedi, M. H. (2006). The Montgomery Äsberg and the Hamilton ratings of depression: A comparison of measures. *European Neuropsychopharmacology*, 16(8), 601–611.

Casey, P., & Doherty, A. (2012). Adjustment disorder: Diagnostic and treatment issues. *Psychiatric Times, 29*, 43–46.

Celio, A. A., Wilfley, D. E., Crow, S. J., Mitchell, J., & Walsh, B. T. (2004). A comparison of the Binge Eating Scale, Questionnaire for Eating and Weight Patterns-Revised, and Eating Disorder Examination Questionnaire with instructions with the Eating Disorder Examination in the assessment of binge eating disorder and its symptoms. *International Journal of Eating Disorders, 36*, 434–444. doi: 10.1002/eat.20057

Center for Adolescent Substance Abuse Research, Children's Hospital Boston. (CEASAR). (2009). *The CRAFFT screening interview*. Retrieved from http://www.ceasar-boston.org/CRAFFT/pdf/CRAFFT_English.pdf

Centers for Disease Control. (CDC). (2005). Mental health in the United States: Prevalence of diagnosis and medication treatment for Attention-deficit/Hyperactivity Disorder—United States, 2003. *Morbidity and Mortality Weekly Report, 54*, 842–847.

Chabrol, H., & Teissedre, F. (2004). Relation between Edinburgh Postnatal Depression Scale scores at 2–3 days and 4–6 weeks postpartum. *Journal of Reproductive and Infant Psychology, 22*(1), 33–39.

Charman, T. (2011). The highs and lows of counting autism. *American Journal of Psychiatry, 168*, 873–875. doi: 10.1176/appi.ajp.2011.11060897

Chiu, S., Webber, M. P., Zeig-Owens, Z., Gustave, J., Lee, R., Kelly, K. J., ... Prezant, D. J. (2011). Performance characteristics of the PTSD Checklist in retired firefighters exposed to the World Trade Center disaster. *Annals of Clinical Psychiatry, 23*, 95–104.

Classen, C., Koopman, C., Hales, R., & Spiegel, D. (1998). Acute stress disorder as a predictor of posttraumatic stress symptoms. *American Journal of Psychiatry, 155*, 620–624.

Clinton, D., & Norring, C. (1999). The Rating of Anorexia and Bulimia (RAB) Interview: Development and preliminary validation. *European Eating Disorders Review, 7*, 362–371.

Coffey, S. F., Dansky, B. S., Falsetti, S. A., Saladin, M. E., & Brady, K. T. (1998). Screening for PTSD in a substance abuse sample: Psychometric properties of a modified version of the PTSD Symptom Scale Self-Report. *Journal of Traumatic Stress, 11*, 393–399.

Coffey, S. F., Gudmundsdottir, B., Beck, J. G., Palyo, S. A., & Miller, L. (2006). Screening for PTSD in motor vehicle accident survivors using the PSS-SR and IES. *Journal of Traumatic Stress, 19*, 119–128. doi: 10.1002/jts.20106

Cole, S. R., Kawachi, I., Maller, S. R., & Berkman, L. F. (2000). Test of item-response bias in the CES-D scale: Experience from the New Haven EPESE Study. *Journal of Clinical Epidemiology, 53*, 285–289.

Connor, K., Davidson, J., Churchill, L., Sherwood, A., Foa, E., & Weisler, R. (2000). Psychometric properties of the Social Phobia Inventory. *British Journal of Psychiatry, 176*, 379–386.

Conybeare, D., Behar, E., Solomon, A., Newman, M. G., & Borkovec, T. D. (2012). The PTSD Checklist—Civilian version: Reliability, validity, and factor structure in a nonclinical sample. *Journal of Clinical Psychology, 68*, 699–713. doi: 10.1002/jclp.21845

Cooper, P. J., Taylor, M. J., Cooper, Z., & Fairburn, C. G. (1987). The development and validation of the Body Shape Questionnaire. *International Journal of Eating Disorders, 6*, 485–494.

Corrigan, P. W. (2007). How clinical diagnosis might exacerbate the stigma of mental illness. *Social Work, 52*, 31–39.

Cotton, M.-A., Ball, C., & Robinson, P. (2003). Four simple questions can help screen for eating disorders. *Journal of General Internal Medicine, 18*, 53–56.

Creamer, M., O'Donnell, M. L., & Pattison, P. (2004). The relationship between acute stress disorder and posttraumatic stress disorder in severely injured trauma survivors. *Behaviour Research and Therapy, 42*, 315–328. doi: 10.1016/S0005-7967(03)00141-4

Creamer, M., Wade, D., Fletcher, S., & Forbes, D. (2011). PTSD among military personnel. *International Review of Psychiatry, 23*, 160–165. doi: 10.3109/09540261.2011.559456

Cuevas, C. A., Bollinger, A. R., Vielhauer, M. J., Morgan, E. E., Sohler, N. L., Brief, D. J., ... Keane, T. M. (2006). HIV/AIDS cost study: Construct validity and factor structure of the PTSD Checklist in dually diagnosed HIV-Seropositive adults. *Journal of Psychological Trauma, 5*, 29–51.

Cummins, L. H., Chan, K. K., Burns, K. M., Blume, A. W., Larimer, M., & Marlatt, G. A. (2003). Validity of the CRAFFT in American-Indian and Alaska-Native adolescents: Screening for drug and alcohol risk. *Journal of Studies on Alcohol, 64*, 727–732.

Daalman, K., Boks, M. P. M., Diederen, K. M. J., de Weijer, A. D., Blom, J. D., Kahn, R. S., & Sommer, I. E. C. (2011). The same or different? A phenomenological comparison of auditory verbal hallucinations in healthy and psychotic individuals. *Journal of Clinical Psychiatry, 72*, 320–325. doi: 10.4088/JCP.09m05797yel

Davis, C. G., Thomas, G., Jesseman, R., & Mazan, R. (2009). Drawing the line on risky use of cannabis: Assessing problematic use with the ASSIST. *Addiction Research and Theory, 17*, 322–332. doi: 10.1080/16066350802334587

Davis, R. A., Flett, G. L., & Besser, A. (2002). Validation of a new scale for measuring problematic Internet use: Implications for pre-employment screening. *CyberPsychology & Behavior, 5*, 331–345.

Dawson, D. A., Grant, B. F., Stinson, F. S., Chou, P. S., Huang, B., & Ruan, W. J. (2005). Recovery from DSM-IV alcohol dependence: United States, 2001–2002. *Addiction, 100*, 281–292. doi: 10.1111/j.1360-0443.2004.00964.x

Dawson, D. A., Grant, B. F., Stinson, F. S., & Zhou, Y. (2005). Effectiveness of the derived Alcohol Use Disorders Identification Test (AUDIT-C) in screening for alcohol use disorders and risk drinking in the US general population. *Alcoholism: Clinical and Experimental Research, 29*, 844–854.

de Jonghe, J. F., & Baneke, J. J. (1989). The Zung Self-Rating Depression Scale: A replication study on reliability, validity, and prediction. *Psychological Reports, 64*, 833–834. doi: 10.2466/pr0.1989.64.3.833

de Meneses-Gaya, C., Zuardi, A. W., Loureiro, S. R., & Crippa, J. A. S. (2009). Alcohol Use Disorders Identification Test (AUDIT): An updated systematic review of psychometric properties. *Psychology & Neuroscience, 2*, 83–97. doi: 10.3922/j.psns.2009.1.12

Demirchyan, A., Petrosyan, V., & Thompson, M. E. (2011). Psychometric value of the Center for Epidemiologic Studies—Depression (CES-D) scale for screening of depressive symptoms in Armenian population. *Journal of Affective Disorders, 133*, 489–498.

Dennis, C. L. (2004). Can we identify mothers at risk for postpartum depression in the immediate postpartum period using the Edinburgh Postnatal Depression Scale? *Journal of Affective Disorders, 78*, 163–169.

Dias, A. M. (2012). The integration of the glutamatergic and the white matter hypotheses of schizophrenia's etiology. *Current Neuropharmacology, 10*, 2–11.

DiGuiseppi, C., Hepburn, S., Davis, J. M., Fidler, D. J., Harway, S., Lee, N. R., ... Robinson, C. (2010). Screening for autism spectrum disorders in children with Down syndrome: Population prevalence and screening test characteristics. *Journal of Developmental and Behavioral Pediatrics, 31*, 181–191. doi: 10.1097/DBP.0b013e3181d5aa6d

Dobie, D. J., Kivlahan, D. R., Maynard, C., Bush, K. R., McFall, M., Epler, A. J., & Bradley, K. A. (2002). Screening for post-traumatic stress disorder in female Veteran's Affairs patients: Validation of the PTSD Checklist. *General Hospital Psychiatry, 24*, 367–374. doi: 10.1016/S0163-8343(02)00207-4

Doninger, G. L., Enders, C. K., & Burnett, K. F. (2005). Validity evidence for Eating Attitudes Test scores in a sample of female college athletes. *Measurement in Physical Education and Exercise Science, 9*, 35–49.

Doyle, S. R., Donovan, D. M., & Kivlahan, D. R. (2007). The factor structure of the Alcohol Use Disorders Identification Test (AUDIT). *Journal of Studies on Alcohol and Drugs, 68*, 474–479.

Drake, R., Haddock, G., Tarrier, N., Bentall, R., & Lewis, S. (2007). The Psychotic Symptom Rating Scales (PSYRATS): Their usefulness and properties in first episode psychosis.

Duffy, M., Gillig, S. E., Tureen, R. M., & Ybarra, M. A. (2002). A critical look at the DSM-IV. *The Journal of Individual Psychology, 58*, 363–373.

Durkin, M. S., Maenner, M. J., Meaney, F. J., Levy, S. E., DiGuiseppi, C., Nicholas, J. S., ... Schieve, L. A. (2010). Socioeconomic inequality in the prevalence of autism spectrum disorder: Evidence from a U.S. cross-sectional study. *PLoS ONE, 5*, 1–8.

Dvir, Y., & Frazier, J. A. (2011). Autism and schizophrenia. *Psychiatric Times, 28*, 34–35.

Dyregrov, A., Mortensen, O., & Dyregrov, K. (2003). Evaluation of a bereavement programme for parents following unexpected child loss. *Tidsskrift for Norsk Psykologforening, 40*, 839–847.

Edmondson, D., Mills, M. A., & Park, C. L. (2010). Factor structure of the Acute Stress Disorder Scale in a sample of Hurricane Katrina evacuees. *Psychological Assessment, 22*, 269–278. doi: 10.1037/a0018506

Edmondson, O. J., Psychogiou, L., Vlachos, H., Netsi, E., & Ramchandani, P. G. (2010). Depression in fathers in the postnatal period: Assessment of the Edinburgh Postnatal Depression Scale as a screening measure. *Journal of Affective Disorders, 125*, 365–368. doi: 10.1016/j.jad.2010.01.069

Edwards, M. C., Cheavens, J. S., Heiy, J. E., & Cukrowicz, K. C. (2010). A reexamination of the factor structure of the Center for Epidemiologic Studies—Depression Scale: Is a one-factor model plausible? *Psychological Assessment, 22*, 711–715. doi: 10.1037/a0019917

Ehlers, A., Bisson, J., Clark, D., Creamer, M., Pilling, S., Richards, D., ... Yule, W. (2010). Do all psychological treatments really work the same in posttraumatic stress disorder? *Clinical Psychology Review, 30*, 269–276. doi: 10.1016/j.cpr.2009.12.001

Ehlers, S., & Gillberg, C. (1993). The epidemiology of Asperger syndrome. A total population study. *Journal of Child Psychology and Psychiatry, 34*, 1327–1350.

Ehlers, S., Gillberg, C., & Wing, L. (1999). A screening questionnaire for Asperger syndrome and other high-functioning autism spectrum disorders in school age children. *Journal of Autism & Developmental Disorders, 29*, 129–141. doi: 10.1023/A:1023040610384

Eldin, A. S., Habib, D., Noufal, A., Farrag, S., Bazaid, K., Al-Sharbati, M...Gaddour, N. (2008). Use of M-CHAT for a multinational screening of young children with autism in the Arab countries. *International Review of Psychiatry, 20*, 281–289. doi: 10.1080/09540260801990324

Englehard, I. M., Arntz, A., & van den Hout, M. A. (2007). Low specificity of symptoms on the post-traumatic stress disorder (PTSD) symptom scale: A comparison of individuals with PTSD, individuals with other anxiety disorders and individuals without psychopathology. *British Journal of Clinical Psychology, 46*, 449–456. doi: 10.1348/014466507X206883

Erford, B. T. (Ed.). (2013). *Assessment for counselors* (2nd ed.). Boston, MA: Cengage.

Esbjorn, B. H., Hoeyer, M., Dyrborg, J., Leth, I., & Kendall, P. C. (2010). Prevalence and co-morbidity among anxiety disorders in a national cohort of psychiatrically referred children and adolescents. *Journal of Anxiety Disorders, 24*, 866–872. doi: 10.1016/j.janxdis.2010.06.009

Evans, C., & Dolan, B. (1993). Body Shape Questionnaire: Derivation of shortened "alternative forms." *International Journal of Eating Disorders, 13*, 315–321.

Falk, D., Yi, H.-Y., & Hiller-Sturmhöfel, S. (2008). An epidemiologic analysis of co-occuring alcohol and drug use and disorders: Findings from the National Epidemiologic Survey of Alcohol and Related Conditions (NESARC). *Alcohol Research & Health, 31*, 100–110.

Falsetti, S. A., Resnick, H. S., Resick, P. A., & Kilpatrick, D. G. (1993). The Modified PTSD Symptom Scale: A brief self-report measure of posttraumatic stress disorder. *The Behavior Therapist, 16*, 161–162.

Fernandez, S., Malacrne, V. L., Wilfley, D. E., & McQuaid, J. (2006). Factor structure of the Bulimia Test—Revised in college women from four ethnic groups. *Cultural Diversity and Ethnic Minority Psychology*, *12*, 403–419. doi: 10.1037/1099-9809.12.3.403

Fiori Nastro, P., Monducci, E., Pappagallo, E., Fagioli, F., Saba, R., Righetti, V., ... Girardi, P. (2010). Prodromal symptoms: A "risk" for patients or psychiatrists? *Clinical Neuropsychiatry: Journal of Treatment Evaluation*, *7*, 49–55.

Foa, E. B., Johnson, K. M., Feeny, N. C., & Treadwell, K. R. H. (2001). The Child PTSD Symptom Scale: A preliminary examination of its psychometric properties. *Journal of Clinical Child Psychology*, *30*, 376–384.

Foa, E. B., Riggs, D. S., Dancu, C. V., & Rothbaum, B. O. (1993). Reliability and validity of a brief instrument for assessing posttraumatic stress disorder. *Journal of Traumatic Stress*, *6*, 459–473. doi: 10.1002/jts.2490060405

Foa, E. B., & Tolin, D. F. (2000). Comparison of the PTSD Symptom Scale—Interview version and the Clinician-Administered PTSD Scale. *Journal of Traumatic Stress*, *13*, 181–191.

Fonseca-Pedrero, E., Sierra-Baigrie, S., Paino, M., Lemos-Giráldez, S., & Muñiz, J. (2011). Factorial structure and measurement invariance of the Bulimic Investigatory Test, Edinburgh across gender and age. *International Journal of Clinical and Health Psychology*, *11*, 109–123.

Fossati, A., Di Ceglie, A., Acquarini, E., Donati, D., Donini, M., Novella, L., & Maffei, C. (2001). The retrospective assessment of childhood attention deficit hyperactivity disorder in adults: Reliability and validity of the Italian version of the Wender Utah Rating Scale. *Comprehensive Psychiatry*, *42*, 326–336.

Freitag, C. M., Retz-Junginger, P., Retz, W., Seitz, C., Palmason, H., Meyer, J., ... von Gontard, A. (2007). German adaptation of the Autism-Spectrum Quotient (AQ): Evaluation and short version AQ-k. *Zeitschrift für Klinische Psychologie und Psychotherapie: Forschung und Praxis*, *36*, 280–289. doi: 10.1026/1616-3443.36.4.280

Fugslang, A. K., Moergeli, H., Hepp-Beg, S., & Schnyder, U. (2002). Who develops acute stress disorder after accidental injuries? *Psychotherapy and Psychosomatics*, *71*, 214–222. doi: 10.1159/000063647

Fuglsang, A. K., Moergeli, H., & Schnyder, U. (2004). Does acute stress disorder predict post-traumatic stress disorder in traffic accident victims? Analysis of a self-report inventory. *Nordic Journal of Psychiatry*, *58*, 223–229. doi: 10.1080/08039480410006278

Gabrys, J. B., & Peters, K. (1985). Reliability, discriminant, and predictive validity of the Zung Self-Rating Depression Scale. *Psychological Reports*, *57*, 1091–1096.

Gallant, J., Storch, E. A., Merlo, L. J., Ricketts, E. D., Geffken, G. R., Goodman, W. K., & Murphy, T. K. (2008). Convergent and discriminant validity of the Children's Yale-Brown Obsessive Compulsive Scale-Symptom Checklist. *Journal of Anxiety Disorders*, *22*, 1369–1376.

Garner, D. M. (2011a). *Interpretation*. Retrieved from http://eat-26.com/interpretation.php

Garner, D. M. (2011b). *Screening and case finding for the general practitioner*. Retrieved from http://eat-26.com/screening.php

Garner, D. M., & Garfinkel, P. E. (1979). The Eating Attitudes Test: An index of the symptoms of anorexia nervosa. *Psychological Medicine*, *9*, 273–279.

Garner, D. M., Olmstead, M. P., Bohr, Y., & Garfinkel, P. E. (1982). The Eating Attitudes Test: Psychometric features and clinical correlates. *Psychological Medicine, 12*, 871–878.

Gauci, M. A., & MacDonald, D. A. (2012). Confirmatory factor analysis of the Posttraumatic Stress Disorder Checklist. *Journal of Aggression, Maltreatment & Trauma, 21*, 321–330. doi: 10.1080/10926771.2012.665429

Ghaderi, A., & Scott, B. (2004). The reliability and validity of the Swedish version of the Body Shape Questionnaire. *Scandinavian Journal of Psychology, 45*, 319–324.

Gillespie, C. F., Bradley, B., Mercer, K., Smith, A. K., Conneely, K., Gapen, M., ... Ressler, K. J. (2009). Trauma exposure and stress-related disorders in inner city primary care patients. *General Hospital Psychiatry, 31*, 505–514. doi: 10.1016/j.genhosppsych.2009.05.003

Goldner, E. M. (2003). Review: Lifetime prevalence of schizophrenia and related disorders is about 5.5 per 1000, but there is significant variation between regions. *Evidence Based Mental Health, 6*, 74–74.

Gong, Y.-X., Liu, J., Li, C.-J., Jia, M.-X., Song, W.-H., & Guo, Y.-Q. (2011). Reliability and validity of the Chinese version of the Modified Checklist for Autism in Toddlers. *Chinese Mental Health Journal, 25*, 409–414.

González, H. M., Tarraf, W., Whitfield, K. E., & Vega, W. A. (2010). The epidemiology of major depression and ethnicity in the United States. *Journal of Psychiatric Research, 44*, 1043–1051.

Gonzalez, J. C., Sanjuán, J., Canete, C., Echánove, M. J., & Leal, C. (2003). Evaluation of auditory hallucinations: The PSYRATS scale. *Actas Españolas De Psiquiatría, 31*, 10–17.

Gormally, J., Black, S., Daston, S., & Rardin, D. (1982). The assessment of binge eating severity among obese persons. *Addictive Behaviors, 7*, 47–55.

Grant, B. F., Stinson, F. S., Dawson, D. A., Chou, S. P., Dufour, M. C., Compton, W., ... Kaplan, K. (2006). Prevalence and co-occurrence of substance use disorders and independent mood and anxiety disorders: Results from the National Epidemiologic Survey on Alcohol and Related Conditions. *Alcohol Research & Health, 29*, 107–120.

Grant, J. D., Vergés, A., Jackson, K. M., Trull, T. J., Sher, K. J., & Bucholz, K. K. (2012). Age and ethnic differences in the onset, persistence and recurrence of alcohol use disorder. *Addiction, 107*, 756–765. doi: 10.1111/j.1360-0443.2011.03721.x

Green, J. (1998). Postnatal depression or perinatal dysphoria? Findings from a longitudinal community-based study using the Edinburgh Postnatal Depression Scale. *Journal of Reproductive and Infant Psychology, 16*, 143–155.

Grubaugh, A. L., Elhai, J. D., Cusack, K. J., Wells, C., & Frueh, B. C. (2007). Screening for PTSD in public-sector mental health settings: The diagnostic utility of the PTSD Checklist. *Depression and Anxiety, 24*, 124–129. doi: 10.1002/da.20226

Guerin, S., Dodd, P., Tyrell, J., McEvoy, J., Buckley, S., & Hillery, J. (2009). An initial assessment of the psychometric properties of the Complicated Grief Questionnaire for People with Intellectual Disabilities (CGQ-ID). *Research in Developmental Disabilities, 30*, 1258–1267. doi: 10.1016/j.ridd.2009.05.002

Haddock, G., McCarron, J., Tarrier, N., & Faragher, E. B. (1999). Scales to measure dimensions of hallucinations and delusions: The Psychotic Symptom Rating Scales (PSYRATS). *Psychological Medicine, 29*, 879–889.

Haddock, G., Wood, L., Watts, R., Dunn, G., Morrison, A. P., & Price, J. (2011). The Subjective Experiences of Psychosis Scale (SEPS): Psychometric evaluation of a scale to assess outcome in psychosis. *Schizophrenia Research, 133*, 244–249. doi: 10.1016/j.schres.2011.09.023

Hamilton, M. (1960). A rating scale for depression. *Journal of Neurology, Neurosurgery & Psychiatry, 23*, 56–62.

Hamrin, V., & Scahill, L. (2004). Acute stress disorder symptoms in gunshot-injured youth. *Journal of Child & Adolescent Psychiatric Nursing, 17*, 161–172.

Harrington, A. (2012). The fall of the schizophrenogenic mother. *The Lancet, 379*, 1292–1293. doi: 10.1016/S0140-6736(12)60546-7

Hatton, C., Haddock, G., Taylor, J. L., Coldwell, J., Crossley, R., & Peckham, N. (2005). The reliability and validity of general psychotic rating scales with people with mild and moderate intellectual disabilities: An empirical investigation. *Journal of Intellectual Disability Research, 49*, 490–500.

Haynes, S. D. (1998). Review of the Eating Inventory. In J. C. Impara & B. S. Plake (Eds.), *The thirteenth mental measurements yearbook*. Retrieved from http://www.buros.unl.edu

Helfricht, S., Landolt, M. A., Moergeli, H., Hepp, U., Wegener, D., & Schnyder, U. (2009). Psychometric evaluation and validation of the German version of the Acute Stress Disorder Scale across two distinct trauma populations. *Journal of Traumatic Stress, 22*, 476–480. doi: 10.1002/jts.20445

Henderson, M., & Freeman, C. P. (1987). A self-rating scale for bulimia: The BITE. *The British Journal of Psychiatry, 150*, 18–24. doi: 10.1192/bjp.150.1.18

Hertzog, C., Van Alstine, J., Usala, P. D., Hultsch, D. F., & Dixon, R. (1990). Measurement properties of the Center for Epidemiologic Studies—Depression Scale (CES-D) in older populations. *Psychological Assessment, 2*, 64–72.

Hides, L., Cotton. S. M., Berger, G., Gleeson, J., O'Donnell, C., Proffitt, T., McGorry, P. D., & Lubman, D. I. (2009). The reliability and validity of the Alcohol, Smoking and Substance Involvement Screening Test (ASSIST) in first-episode psychosis. *Addictive Behaviors, 34*, 821–825. doi: 10.1016/j.addbeh.2009.03.001

Hill, L. S., Reid, F., Morgan, J. F., & Lacey, J. H. (2010). SCOFF: The development of an eating disorder screening questionnaire. *International Journal of Eating Disorders, 43*, 344–351. doi: 10.1002/eat.20679

Hirschel, M. J., & Schulenberg, S. E. (2010). On the viability of PTSD Checklist (PCL) short form use: Analyses from Mississippi Gulf Coast Hurricane Katrina survivors. *Psychological Assessment, 22*, 460–464. doi: 10.1037/a0018336

Hirschfeld, R. M., Williams, J. B., Spitzer, R. L., Calabrese, J. R., Flynn, L., Keck, P. E., ... Zajecka, J. (2000). Development and validation of a screening instrument for bipolar spectrum disorder: The Mood Disorder Questionnaire. *American Journal of Psychiatry, 157*, 1873–1875. doi: 10.1176/appi.ajp.157.11.1873

Hoek, H. W., & van Hoeken, D. (2003). Review of the prevalence and incidence of eating disorders. *International Journal of Eating Disorders, 34*, 383–396. doi: 10.1002/eat.10222

Hoekstra, R. A., Bartels, M., Cath, D. C., & Boomsma, D. I. (2008). Factor structure, reliability and criterion validity of the Autism-Spectrum Quotient (AQ): A study in Dutch population and patient groups. *Journal of Autism and Developmental Disorders, 38*, 1555–1566. doi: 10.1007/s10803-008-0538-x

Hoekstra, R. A., Vinkhuyzen, A. A. E., Wheelwright, S., Bartels, M., Boomsma, D. I., Baron-Cohen, S., ... van der Sluis, S. (2011). The construction and validation of an abridged version of the Autism-Spectrum Quotient (AQ-Short). *Journal of Autism and Developmental Disorders, 41*, 589–596. doi: 10.1007/s10803-010-1073-0

Hudson, J. I., Hiripi, E., Pope, H. G., Jr., & Kessler, R. C. (2007). The prevalence and correlates of eating disorders in the national comorbidity survey replication. *Biological Psychiatry, 61*, 348–358. doi: 10.1016/j.biopsych.2006.03.040

Humeniuk, R., Ali, R., Babor, T. F., Farrell, M., Formigoni, M. L., Jittiwutikarn, J., ... Simon, S. (2008). Validation of the Alcohol, Smoking and Substance Involvement Screening Test (ASSIST). *Addiction, 103*, 1039–1047. doi: 10.1111/j.1360-0443.2007.02114.x

Hurst, R. M., Mitchell, J. T., Kimbrel, N. A., Kwapil, T. K., & Nelson-Gray, R. O. (2007). Examination of the reliability and factor structure of the Autism Spectrum Quotient (AQ) in a non-clinical sample. *Personality and Individual Differences, 43*, 1938–1949. doi: 10.1016/j.paid.2007.06.012

Inada, N., Koyama, T., Inokuchi, E., Kuroda, M., & Kamio, Y. (2011). Reliability and validity of the Japanese version of the Modified Checklist for Autism in Toddlers (M-CHAT). *Research in Autism Spectrum Disorders, 5*, 330–336. doi: 10.1016/j.rasd.2010.04.016

Ising, H. K., Veling, Q., Loewy, R. L., Rietveld, M. W., Rietdijk, J., Dragt, S., ... van der Gaag, M. (2012). The validity of the 16-item version of the Prodromal Questionnaire (PQ-16) to screen for ultra-high risk of developing psychosis in the general help-seeking population. *Schizophrenia Bulletin, 38*, 1–9. doi: 10.1093/schbul/sbs068

Israelski, D. M., Prentiss, D. E., Lubega, S., Balmas, G., Garcia, P., Muhammad, M., ... Koopman, C. (2007). Psychiatric co-morbidity in vulnerable populations receiving primary care for HIV/AIDS. *AIDS Care, 19*, 220–225. doi: 10.1080/0954012600774230

Jarrett, M., Craig, T., Parrott, J., Forrester, A., Winton-Brown, T., Maguire, H., ... Valmaggia, L. (2012). Identifying men at ultra high risk of psychosis in a prison population. *Schizophrenia Research, 136*, 1–6. doi: 10.1016/j.schres.2012.01.025

Ji, S., Long, Q., Newport, D. J., Na, H., Knight, B., Zach, E. B., ... Stowe, Z. N. (2011). Validity of depression rating scales during pregnancy and the postpartum period: Impact of trimester and parity. *Journal of Psychiatric Research, 45*, 213–219.

Jia, R., & Jia, H. H. (2009). Factorial validity of problematic Internet use scales. *Computers in Human Behavior, 25*, 1335–1342. doi: 10.1016/j.chb.2009.06.004

Jorm, A. F. (2011). "Prodromal diagnosis" of psychosis: An impartial commentary. *Australian & New Zealand Journal of Psychiatry, 45*, 520–523. doi: 10.3109/00048674.2011.585132

Jung, S. M., Kim, M. K., Lee, J. B., Choi, J. H., Jung, B. J., & Byun, W. T. (2007). Reliability and validity of the Korean version of the Psychotic Symptom Rating Scale. *Journal of the Korean Neuropsychiatric Association, 46*, 201–213.

Kangas, M., Henry, J. L., & Bryant, R. A. (2005). The course of psychological disorders in the 1st year after cancer diagnosis. *Journal of Consulting and Clinical Psychology, 73*, 763–768. doi: 10.1037/0022-006X.73.4.763

Karlsson, J., Persson, L. O., Sjöström, L., & Sullivan, M. (2000). Psychometric properties and factor structure of the Three-Factor Eating Questionnaire (TFEQ) in obese men and women: Results from the Swedish Obese Subjects (SOS) study. *International Journal of Obesity, 24*, 1715–1725.

Kaufman, J., Birmaher, B., Brent, D., Rao, U., Flynn, C., Moreci, P., ... Ryan, N. (1997). Schedule for Affective Disorders and Schizophrenia for School-Age Children—Present and Lifetime Version (K-SADS-PL): Initial reliability and validity data. *Journal of the American Academy of Child & Adolescent Psychiatry, 36*, 980–998.

Kelly, T. M., Donovan, J. E., Chung, T., Bukstein, O. G., & Cornelius, J. R. (2009). Brief screens for detecting alcohol use disorder among 18–20 year old young adults in emergency departments: Comparing AUDIT-C, CRAFFT, RAPS4-QF, FAST, RUFT-Cut, and DSM-IV 2-Item Scale. *Addictive Behaviors, 34*, 668–674. doi: 10.1016/j.addbeh.2009.03.038

Kersting, A., Brahler, E., Glaesmer, H., & Wagner, B. (2011). Prevalence of complicated grief in a representative population-based sample. *Journal of Affective Disorders, 131*, 339–343. doi: 10.1016/j.jad.2010.11.032

Kersting, A., & Kroker, K. (2010). Prolonged grief as a distinct disorder, specifically affecting female health. *Archives of Women's Mental Health, 13*, 27–28. doi: 10.1007/s00737-009-0112-3

Keski-Rahkonen, A., Hoek, H. W., Susser, E. S., Linna, M. S., Sihvola, E., Raevuori, A, ... Rissanen, A. (2007). Epidemiology and course of anorexia nervosa in the community. *American Journal of Psychiatry, 164*, 1259–1265.

Kessler, R. C., Adler, L., Barkley, R., Biederman, J., Conners, C. K., Demler, O., ... Zaslavsky, A. M. (2006). The prevalence and correlates of adult AD/HD in the United States: Results from the National Comorbidity Survey Replication. *American Journal of Psychiatry, 163*, 716–723. doi: 10.1176/appi.ajp.163.4.716

Kessler, R. C., Adler, L. A., Gruber, M. J., Sarawate, C. A., Spencer, T., & Van Brunt, D. L. (2007). Validity of the World Health Organization Adult AD/HD Self-Report Scale (ASRS) Screener in a representative sample of health plan members. *International Journal of Methods in Psychiatric Research, 16*(2), 52–65.

Kessler, R. C., Berglund, P., Demler, O., Jin, R., Koretz, D., & Merikangas, K. R. (2003). The epidemiology of major depressive disorder: Results from the National Comorbidity Survey Replication (NCS-R). *Journal of the American Medical Association, 289*(23), 3095–3105.

Kessler, R. C., Berglund, P., Demler, O., Jin, R., Merikangas, K. R., & Walters, E. E. (2005). Lifetime prevalence and age-of-onset distributions of DSM-IV disorders in the National Comorbidity Survey Replication. *Archives of General Psychiatry, 62*, 593–602.

Kessler, R. C., Chiu, W. T., Demler, O., & Walters, E. E. (2005). Prevalence, severity, and comorbidity of twelve-month DSM-IV disorders in the National Comorbidity Survey Replication (NCS-R). *Archives of General Psychiatry, 62*, 617–627.

Kessler, R. C., Coccaro, E. F., Fava, M., Jaeger, S., Jin, R., & Walters, E. (2006). The prevalence and correlates of DSM-IV Intermittent Explosive Disorder in the National Comorbidity Survey Replication. *Archives of General Psychiatry, 63*, 669–678. doi: 10.1001/archpsyc.63.6.669

Kim, S. E., Jung, H. Y., Hwang, S. S., Chang, J. S., Kim, Y., Ahn, Y. M., & Kim, Y. S. (2010). The usefulness of a self-report questionnaire measuring auditory verbal hallucinations. *Progress in Neuro-Psychopharmacology and Biological Psychiatry, 34*, 968–973. doi: /10.1016/j.pnpbp.2010.05.005

Kim, Y. S., Leventhal, B. L., Koh, Y.-J., Fombonne, E., Laska, E., Lim, E.-C., ... Grinker, R. R. (2011). Prevalence of autism spectrum disorders in a total population sample. *American Journal of Psychiatry, 168*, 904–912. doi: 10.1176/appi.ajp.2011.10101532

King, B. H., & Lord, C. (2010). Is schizophrenia on the autism spectrum? *Brain Research, 1380*, 34–41. doi: 10.1016/j.brainres.2010.11.031

King, L. C., & Werner, P. D. (2012). Attachment, social support, and responses following the death of a companion animal. *Omega, 64*, 119–141.

Kitamura T., Hirano, H., Chen, Z., & Hirata, M. (2004). Factor structure of the Zung Self-Rating Depression Scale in first-year university students in Japan. *Psychiatry Research, 128, 281–289.*

Kleinman, J. M., Robins, D. L., Ventola, P. E., Pandey, J., Boorstein, H. C., Esser, E. L., ... Fein, D. (2008). The Modified Checklist for Autism in Toddlers: A follow-up study investigating the early detection of autism spectrum disorders. *Journal of Autism & Developmental Disorders, 38*, 827–839. doi: 10.1007/s10803-007-0450-9

Kleinman, J. M., Ventola, P. E., Pandey, J., Verbalis, A. D., Barton, M., Hodgson, S., ... Fein, D. (2008). Diagnostic stability in very young children with autism spectrum disorders. *Journal of Autism & Developmental Disorders, 38*, 606–615. doi: 10.1007/s10803-007-0427-8

Kloosterman, P. H., Keefer, K. V., Kelley, E. A., Summerfeldt, L. J., & Parker, J. D. (2011). Evaluation of the factor structure of the Autism-Spectrum Quotient. *Personality and Individual Differences, 50*, 310–314. doi: 10.1016/j.paid.2010.10.015

Knight, J. R., Harris, S. K., Sherrit, L., Van Hook, S., Lawrence, N., Brooks, T., ... Kulig, J. (2007). Adolescents' preference for substance abuse screening in primary care practice. *Substance Abuse, 28*, 107–117. doi: 10.1300/J465v28n04_03

Knight, J. R., Sherritt, L., Harris, S. K., Gates, E. C., & Chang, G. (2003). Validity of brief alcohol screening tests among adolescents: A comparison of the AUDIT, POSIT, CAGE, and CRAFFT. *Alcoholism: Clinical and Experimental Research, 27*, 67–73. doi: 10.1097/00000374-200301000-00012

Knight, J. R., Sherritt, L., Shrier, L. A., Harris, S. K., & Chang, G. (2002). Validity of the CRAFFT substance abuse screening test among adolescent clinic patients. *Archives of Pediatrics & Adolescent Medicine, 156*, 607–614.

Knight, R. G., Williams, S., McGee, R., & Olaman, S. (1997). Psychometric properties of the Center for Epidemiologic Studies—Depression Scale (CES-D) in a sample of women in middle life. *Behaviour Research and Therapy, 35*, 373–380.

Kocabaşoğlu, N., Özdemir, A. C., Yargiç, I., & Geyran, P. (2005). The validity and safety of Turkish PTSD Checklist—Civilian version (PCL-C) scale. *Yeni Symposium: Psikiyatri, nöroloji ve davraniş bilimleri dergisi, 43*, 126–134.

Koch, E., Schultze-Lutter, F., Schimmelmann, B. G., & Resch, F. (2010). On the importance and detection of prodromal symptoms from the perspective of child and adolescent psychiatry. *Clinical Neuropsychiatry: Journal of Treatment Evaluation, 7*, 38–48.

Kokotailo, P. K. (2004). Validity of the Alcohol Use Disorders Identification Test in college students. *Alcoholism: Clinical & Experimental Research, 28*, 914–920.

Koopman, C., Zarcone, J., Mann, M., Freinkel, A., & Spiegel, D. (1998). Acute stress reactions of psychiatry staff to a threatening patient. *Journal of Anxiety, Stress and Coping, 11*, 27–45.

Kopp, S., & Gillberg, C. (2011). The Autism Spectrum Screening Questionnaire (ASSQ)–Revised Extended Version (ASSQ-REV): An instrument for better capturing the autism phenotype in girls? A preliminary study involving 191 clinical cases and community controls. *Research in Developmental Disabilities, 32*, 2875–2888. doi: 10.1016/j.ridd.2011.05.017

Koran, L. M., Abujaoude, E., Large, M. D., & Serpe, R. T. (2008). The prevalence of Body Dysmorphic Disorder in the United States adult population. *CNS Spectrums, 13*, 316–322.

Kormas, G., Critselis, E., Janikian, M., Kafetzis, D., & Tsitskia, A. (2011). Risk factors and psychosocial characteristics of potential problematic and problematic Internet use among adolescents: A cross-sectional study. *BMC Public Health, 11*, 595–602.

Köse, S., Bora, E., Erermiş, S., & Aydın, C. (2010). Psychometric features of Turkish version of Autism-Spectrum Quotient. *Anadolu Psikiyatri Dergisi, 11*, 253–260.

Koslowsky, M., Scheinberg, Z., Bleich, A., Mark, M., Apter, A., Danon, Y., & Solomon, Z. (1992). The factor structure and criterion validity of the short form of the Eating Attitudes Test. *Journal of Personality Assessment, 58*, 27–35.

Kozlowski, A. M., Matson, J. L., Worley, J. A., Sipes, M., & Horovitz, M. (2012). Defining characteristics for young children meeting cutoff on the Modified Checklist for Autism in Toddlers. *Research in Autism Spectrum Disorders, 6*, 472–479. doi: 10.1016/j.rasd.2011.07.007

Kriston, L., & von Wolff, A. (2011). Not as golden as standards should be: Interpretation of the Hamilton Rating Scale for Depression. *Journal of Affective Disorders, 128*(1–2), 175–177.

Kronmüller, K.-T., von Bock, A., Grupe, S., Büche, L., Gentner, N. C., Rückl, S., ... Mundt, C. (2011). Psychometric evaluation of the Psychotic Symptom Rating Scales. *Comprehensive Psychiatry, 52*, 102–108. doi: 10.1016/j.comppsych.2010.04.014

Kurita, H., Koyama, T., & Osada, H. (2005). Autism-Spectrum Quotient–Japanese version and its short forms for screening normally intelligent persons with pervasive developmental disorders. *Psychiatry and Clinical Neurosciences, 59*, 490–496.

Kuss, D. J., & Griffiths, M. D. (2011). Online social networking and addiction: A review of the psychological literature. *International Journal of Environmental Research and Public Health, 8*, 3528–3552. doi: 10.3390/ijerph8093528

Lähteenmäki, S., Aalto-Setälä, T., Suokas, J. T., Saarni, S. E., Perälä, J., Saarni, S., ... Suvisaari, J. M. (2009). Validation of the Finnish version of the SCOFF questionnaire among young adults aged 20 to 35 years. *BMC Psychiatry, 9*, 5–12. doi: 10.1186/1471-244X-9-5

Landolt, M., Boehler, U., Schwager, C., Schallberger, U., & Nuessli, R. (1998). Post-traumatic stress disorder in paediatric patients and their parents: An exploratory study. *Journal of Paediatric Child Health, 34*, 539–543.

Lang, A. J., & Stein, M. B. (2005). An abbreviated PTSD Checklist for use as a screening instrument in primary care. *Behaviour Research & Therapy, 43*, 585–594. doi: 10.1016/j.brat.2004.04.005

Lee, J. J., Kim, K. W., Kim, T. H., Park, J. H., Lee, S. B., Park, J. W., ... Steffens, D. C. (2011). Cross-cultural considerations in administrating the Center for Epidemiologic Studies–Depression Scale. *Gerontology, 57*, 455–461. doi: 10.1159/000318030.

Lee, S. W., Stewart, S. M., Striegel-Moore, R. H., Lee, S., Ho, S.-Y., Lee, P. W. H., ... Lam, T.-H. (2007). Validation of the Eating Disorder Diagnostic Scale for use with Hong Kong adolescents. *International Journal of Eating Disorders, 40*, 569–574. doi: 10.1002/eat.20413

Lefkowitz, D. S., Baxt., C., & Evans, J. R. (2010). Prevalence and correlates of posttraumatic stress and postpartum depression in parents of infants in the neonatal intensive care unit (NICU). *Journal of Clinical Psychology in Medical Settings, 17*, 230–237. doi: 10.1007/s10880-010-9202-7

Leibson, C. L., Katusic, S. K., Barbaresi, W. J., Ransom, J., & O'Brien, P. C. (2001). Use and costs of medical care for children and adolescents with and without attention-deficit/hyperactivity disorder. *The Journal of the American Medical Association, 285*(1), 60–66.

Leonard, H., Dixon, G., Whitehouse, A. J. O., Bourke, J., Aiberti, K., Nassar, N., ... Glasson, E. J. (2010). Unpacking the complex nature of the autism epidemic. *Research in Autism Spectrum Disorders, 4*, 548–554. doi: 10.1016/j.rasd.2010.01.003

Lepage, J.-F., Lortie, M., Taschereau-Dumouchel, V., & Theoret, H. (2009). Validation of the French-Canadian versions of the Empathy Quotient and Autism Spectrum Quotient. *Canadian Journal of Behavioural Science, 41*, 272–276. doi: 10.1037/a0016248

Levy, S., Sherritt, L., Harris, S. K., Gates, E. C., Holder, D. W., Kulig, J. W., & Knight, J. R. (2004). Test-retest reliability of adolescents' self-report of substance use. *Alcoholism: Clinical and Experimental Research, 28*, 1236–1241. doi: 10.1097/01.ALC.0000134216.22162.A5

Lewinsohn, P. M., Rohde, P., & Farrington, D. P. (2000). The OADP-CDS: A brief screener for adolescent conduct disorder. *Journal of the American Academy of Child and Adolescent Psychiatry, 39*, 888–895.

Li, H., Wang, L., Shi, Z., Zhang, Y., Wu, K., & Liu, P. (2011). Diagnostic utility of the PTSD Checklist in detecting PTSD in Chinese earthquake victims. *Psychological Reports, 107*, 733–739. doi: 10.2466/03.15.20.PR0.107.6.733-739

Li, Z., & Hicks, M. H. R. (2010). The CES-D in Chinese American women: Construct validity, diagnostic validity for major depression, and cultural response bias. *Psychiatry Research, 175*, 227–232.

Liu, T. C., Desai, R. A., Krishnan-Sarin, S., Cavallo, D. A., & Potenza, M. N. (2011). Problematic Internet use and health in adolescents: Data from a high school survey in Connecticut. *Journal of Clinical Psychiatry, 72*, 836–845. doi: 10.4088/JCP.10m06057

Liu, T. C., & Potenza, M. N. (2007). Problematic Internet use: Clinical implications. *CNS Spectrums, 12*, 453–466.

Lobo, A., Chamorro, L., Luque, A., & Dal-Ré, R. (2001). Validation into Spanish of the Hamilton Anxiety Rating Scale (HARS) and the Montgomery-Asberg Depression Rating Scale (MADRS). *European Neuropsychopharmacology, 11*, 346–347.

Loewy, R. L., Bearden, C. E., Johnson, J. K., Raine, A., & Cannon, T. D. (2005). The Prodromal Questionnaire (PQ): Preliminary validation of a self-report screening measure for prodromal and psychotic symptoms. *Schizophrenia Research, 77*, 141–149. doi: 10.1016/j.schres.2005.02.009

Loewy, R. L., Johnson, J. K., & Cannon, T. D. (2007). Self-report of attenuated psychotic experiences in a college population. *Schizophrenia Research, 93*, 144–151. doi: 10.1016/j.schres.2007.02.010

Loewy, R. L., Pearson, R. P., Vinogradov, S., Bearden, C. E., & Cannon, T. D. (2011). Psychosis risk screening with the Prodromal Questionnaire–Brief Version (PQ-B). *Schizophrenia Research, 129*, 42–46. doi: 10.1016/j.schres.2011.03.029

Loewy, R. L., Therman, S., Manninen, M., Huttunen, M. O., & Cannon, T. D. (2012). Prodromal psychosis screening in adolescent psychiatry clinics. *Early Intervention in Psychiatry, 6*, 69–75. doi: 10.1111/j.1751-7893.2011.00286.x

Löwe, B., Decker, O., Müller, S., Brähler, E., Schellberg, D., Herzog, W., & Herzberg, P. (2008). Validation and standardization of the Generalized Anxiety Disorder Screener (GAD-7) in the general population. *Medical Care, 46*, 266–274. doi: 10.1097/MLR.0b013e318160d093

Lublin, H., Eberhard, J., & Levander, S. (2005). Current therapy issues and unmet clinical needs in the treatment of schizophrenia: A review of the new generation antipsychotics. *International Clinical Psychopharmacology, 20*, 183–198. doi: 10.1097/00004850-200507000-00001

Luyster, R. J., Kuban, K. C. K., O'Shea, T. M., Paneth, N., Allred, E. N., & Leviton, A. (2011). The Modified Checklist for Autism in Toddlers in extremely low gestational age newborns: Individual items associated with motor, cognitive, vision and hearing limitations. *Paediatric & Perinatal Epidemiology, 25*, 366–376. doi: 10.1111/j.1365-3016.2010.01187.x

Mackin, R. S., & Horner, M. D. (2005). Relationship of the Wender Utah Rating Scale to objective measures of attention. *Comprehensive Psychiatry, 46*, 468–471.

Magruder, K. M., & Yeager, D. E. (2009). The prevalence of PTSD across war eras and the effect of deployment on PTSD: A systematic review and meta-analysis. *Psychiatric Annals, 39*, 778–788.

Maier, W., Buller, R., Philipp, M., & Heuser, I. (1988). The Hamilton Anxiety Scale: Reliability, validity and sensitivity to change in anxiety and depressive disorders. *Journal of Affective Disorders, 14*, 61–68.

Manne, S. L., Du Hamel, K., Gallelli, K., Sorgen, K., & Redd, W. H. (1998). Posttraumatic stress disorder among mothers of pediatric cancer survivors: Diagnosis, comorbidity, and utility of the PTSD Checklist as a screening instrument. *Journal of Pediatric Psychology, 23*, 357–366.

Margiotta, S. M., Anastas, J. W., Stamm, B. H., & Everett, J. (1999). Effects of person-under-train (PUT) incidents on locomotive engineers. Paper presented at the 14th Annual Conference of the International Society for Traumatic Stress Studies, Miami, FL.

Mattila, M.-L., Jussila, K., Kuusikko, S., Kielinen, M., Linna, S.-L., Ebeling, H., ... Moilanen, I. (2009). When does the Autism Spectrum Screening Questionnaire (ASSQ) predict autism spectrum disorders in primary school-aged children? *European Child & Adolescent Psychiatry, 18*, 499–509. doi: 10.1007/s00787-009-0044-5

Maughan, B., Rowe, R., Messer, J., Goodman, R., & Meltzer, H. (2004). Conduct disorder and oppositional defiant disorder in a national sample: Developmental epidemiology. *Journal of Child Psychology & Psychiatry, 45*, 609–621. doi: 10.1111/j.1469-7610.2004.00250.x

Mazzeo, S. E. (1999). Modification of an existing measure of body image preoccupation and its relationship to disordered eating in female college students. *Journal of Counseling Psychology, 46*, 42–50.

Mazzeo, S. E., Aggen, S. H., Anderson, C., Tozzi, F., & Bulik, C. M. (2003). Investigating the structure of the Eating Inventory (Three-Factor Eating Questionnaire): A confirmatory approach. *International Journal of Eating Disorders, 34,* 255–264. doi: 10.1002/eat.10180

McCabe, S. E., West, B. T., Teter, C. J., Cranford, J. A., Ross-Durow, P. L., & Boyd, C. J. (2012). Adolescent nonmedical users of prescription opioids: Brief screening and substance use disorders. *Addictive Behaviors, 37.* doi: 10.1016/j.addbeh.2012.01.021

McCann, B. S., Scheele, L., Ward, N., & Roy-Byrne, P. (2000). Discriminant validity of the Wender Utah Rating Scale for Attention-Deficit/Hyperactivity Disorder in adults. *The Journal of Neuropsychiatry and Clinical Neurosciences, 12,* 240–245. doi: 10.1176/appi.neuropsych.12.2.240

McCarthy, D. M., Simmons, J. R., Smith, G. T., Tomlinson, K. L., & Hill, K. K. (2002). Reliability, stability, and factor structure of the Bulimia Test—Revised and Eating Disorder Inventory—2 scales in adolescence. *Assessment, 9,* 382–389. doi: 10.1177/1073191102238196

McDonald, S. D., & Calhoun, P. S. (2010). The diagnostic accuracy of the PTSD Checklist: A critical review. *Clinical Psychology Review, 30,* 976–987. doi: 10.1016/j.cpr.2010.06.012

McLean, C. P., Asnaani, A., Litz, B. T., & Hofmann, S. G. (2010). Gender differences in anxiety disorders: Prevalence, course of illness, comorbidity and burden of illness. *Journal of Anxiety Disorders, 24,* 866–872. doi:10.1016/j.janxids.2010.06.009

Meerkerk, G.-J., van der Eijnden, R. J. J. M., Vermulst, A. A., & Garretsen, H. F. L. (2009). The Compulsive Internet Use Scale (CIUS): Some psychometric properties. *CyberPsychology & Behavior, 12,* 1–6. doi: 10.1089/cpb.2008.0181

Meiser-Stedman, R., Yule, W., Smith, P., Glucksman, E. & Dalgleish, T. (2005). Acute stress disorder and posttraumatic stress disorder in children and adolescents involved in assaults or motor vehicle accidents. *The American Journal of Psychiatry, 162,* 1381–1383. doi: 10.1176/appi.ajp.162.7.1381

Melhem, N. M., Moritz, G., Walker, M., Shear, K., & Brent, D. (2007). Phenomenology and correlates of complicated grief in children and adolescents. *Journal of the American Academy of Child & Adolescent Psychiatry, 46,* 493–499. doi: 10.1097/chi.0b013e31803062a9

Merikangas, K. R., He, J., Burstein, M., Swanson, S. A., Avenevoli, S., Cui, L., ... Swendsen, J. (2010). Lifetime prevalence of mental disorders in U.S. adolescents: Results from the National Comorbidity Study—Adolescent Supplement (NCS-A). *Journal of the American Academy of Child and Adolescent Psychiatry, 49,* 980–989.

Miles, H., Winstock, A., & Strang, J. (2001). Identifying young people who drink too much: The clinical utility of the five-item Alcohol Use Disorders Identification Test. *Drug and Alcohol Review, 20,* 9–18. doi: 10/108009595230020029347

Mintz, L. B., & O'Halloran, M. S. (2000). The Eating Attitudes Test: Validation with DSM-IV eating disorder criteria. *Journal of Personality Assessment, 74,* 489–503.

Mitchell, A. M., Kim, Y., Prigerson, H. G., & Mortimer-Stephens, M. (2004). Complicated grief in survivors of suicide. *Crisis, 25,* 12–18. doi: 10.1027/0227-5910.25.1.12

Mitka, M. (2010). Rising autism rates still pose a mystery. *Journal of the American Medical Association, 303,* 602.

Mond, J. M., Myers, T. C., Crosby, R. D., Hay, P. J., Rodgers, B., Morgan, J. F., ... Mitchell, J. E. (2008). Screening for eating disorders in primary care: EDE-Q versus SCOFF. *Behaviour Research and Therapy*, *46*, 612–622. doi: 10.1016/j.brat.2008.02.003

Morcillo, C., Duarte, C. S., Sala, R., Wang, S., Lejuez, C. W., Kerridge, B. T., & Blanco, C. (2012). Conduct disorder and adult psychiatric diagnoses: Associations and gender differences in the U.S. adult population. *Journal of Psychiatric Research*, *46*, 323–330.

Morgan, J. F., Reid, F., & Lacey, J. H. (1999). The SCOFF questionnaire: Assessment of a new screening tool for eating disorders. *British Medical Journal*, *319*, 1467–1468.

Morgan, V. A., Valuri, G. M., Croft, M. L., Griffith, J. A., Shah, S., Young, D. J., & Jablensky, A. V. (2011). Cohort profile: Pathways of risk from conception to disease: The western Australian schizophrenia high-risk e-cohort. *International Journal of Epidemiology*, *40*, 1477–1485. doi: 10.1093/ije/dyq167

Morojele, N. K., Saban, A., & Seedat, S. (2012). Clinical presentations and diagnostic issues in dual diagnosis disorders. *Current Opinion in Psychiatry*, *25*, 181–186.

Morrison, A. K. (2009). Cognitive behavior therapy for people with schizophrenia. *Psychiatry*, *6*, 32–39.

Mottram, P., Wilson, K., & Copeland, J. (2000). Validation of the Hamilton Depression Rating Scale and Montgomery and Asberg Rating Scales in terms of AGECAT depression cases. *International Journal of Geriatric Psychiatry*, *15*, 1113–1119.

MTA Cooperative Group. (1999a). A 14-month randomized clinical trial of treatment strategies for attention-deficit/hyperactivity disorder: The MTA Cooperative Group. Multimodal Treatment Study of Children with AD/HD. *Archives of General Psychiatry*, *56*, 1073–1086.

MTA Cooperative Group. (1999b). Moderators and mediators of treatment response for children with attention-deficit/hyperactivity disorder: The Multimodal Treatment Study of children with attention-deficit/hyperactivity disorder. *Archives of General Psychiatry*, *56*, 1088–1096.

Mueser, K. T., Rosenberg, S. D., Fox, L., Salyers, M. P., Ford, J. D., & Carty, P. (2001). Psychometric evaluation of trauma and posttraumatic stress disorder assessments in persons with severe mental illness. *Psychological Assessment*, *13*, 110–117. doi: 10.1037/1040-3590.13.1.110

Nacasch, N., Foa, E. B., Huppert, J. D., Tzur, D., Fostick, L., Dinstein, Y., ... Zohar, J. (2011). Prolonged exposure therapy for combat- and terror-related posttraumatic stress disorder: A randomized control comparison with treatment as usual. *Journal of Clinical Psychiatry*, *72*, 1174–1180. doi: 10.4088/JCP.09m05682blu

Naifeh J. A., Elhai, J. D., Kashdan, T. B., & Grubaugh, A. L. (2008). The PTSD Symptom Scale's latent structure: An examination of trauma-exposed medical patients. *Journal of Anxiety Disorders*, *22*, 1355–1368. doi: 10.1016/j.janxdis.2008.01.016

Nalwa, K., & Anand, A. P. (2003). Internet addiction in students: A cause of concern. *CyberPsychology & Behavior*, *6*, 653–656.

Nauta, M. H., Scholing, A., Rapee, R. M., Abbott, M., Spence, S. H. & Waters, A. (2004). A parent report measure of children's anxiety. *Behaviour Research and Therapy*, *42*, 813–839.

Nevonen, L., Broberg, A. G., Clinton, D., & Norring, C. (2003). A measure for the assessment of eating disorders: Reliability and validity studies of the Rating of Anorexia and Bulimia Interview–Revised version (RAB-R). *Scandinavian Journal of Psychology*, *44*, 303–310.

Newcombe, D. A. L., Humeniuk, R. E., & Ali, R. (2005). Validation of the World Health Organization Alcohol, Smoking and Substance Involvement Screening Test (ASSIST): Report of results from the Australian site. *Drug and Alcohol Review*, *24*, 217–226. doi: 10.1080/09595230500170266

Noma, S., Nakai, Y., Hamagaki, S., Uehara, M., Hayashi, A., & Hayashi, T. (2006). Comparison between the SCOFF questionnaire and the Eating Attitudes Test in patients with eating disorders. *International Journal of Psychiatry in Clinical Practice*, *10*, 27–32. doi: 10.1080/13651500500305275

Norman, S. B., Campbell-Sills, L., Hitchcock, C. A., Sullivan, S., Rochlin, A., Wilkins, K. C., & Stein, M. B. (2011). Psychometrics of a brief measure of anxiety to detect severity and impairment: The Overall Anxiety Severity and Impairment Scale (OASIS). *Journal of Psychiatric Research*, *45*, 262–268.

Norris, M., & Lecavalier, L. (2010). Screening accuracy of level 2 autism spectrum disorder rating scales: A review of selected instruments. *Autism*, *14*, 263–284. doi: 10.1177/1362361309348071

Ocker, L. B., Lam, E. T. C., Jensen, B. E., & Zhang, J. J. (2007). Psychometric properties of the Eating Attitudes Test. *Measurement in Physical Education and Exercise Science*, *11*, 25–48.

O'Donnell, M. L., Creamer, M., Bryant, R. A., Schnyder, U., & Shalev, A. (2003). Posttraumatic disorders following injury: An empirical and methodological review. *Clinical Psychology Review*, *23*, 587–603. doi: 10.1016/S0272-7358(03)00036-9

Ott, C. H. (2003). The impact of complicated grief on mental and physical health at various points in the bereavement process. *Death Studies*, *27*, 249–272. doi: 10.1080/07481180390137044

Özcan, N. K., & Buzlu, S. (2005). An assistive tool in determining problematic Internet use: Validity and reliability of the "Online Cognition Scale" in a sample of university students. *Bağimlik Dergisi*, *6*, 19–26.

Özcan, N. K., & Buzlu, S. (2007). Internet use and its relation with the psychosocial situation for a sample of university students. *CyberPsychology & Behavior*, *10*, 767–772. doi: 10.1089/cpb.2007.9953

Ozer, E. J., Best, S. R., Lipsey, T. L., & Weiss, D. S. (2008). Predictors of posttraumatic stress disorder and symptoms in adults: A meta-analysis. *Psychological Trauma: Theory, Research, Practice, and Policy*, *S*, 3–36. doi: 10.1037/1942-9681.S.1.3

Palmieri, P. A., Weathers, F. W., Difede, J., & King, D. W. (2007). Confirmatory factor analysis of the PTSD Checklist and the Clinician-Administered PTSD Scale in disaster workers exposed to the world trade center ground zero. *Journal of Abnormal Psychology*, *116*, 329–341. doi: 10.1037/0021-843X.116.2.329

Pancheri, P., Picardi, A., Pasquini, M., Gaetano, P., & Biondi, M. (2002). Psychopathological dimensions of depression: A factor study of the 17-item Hamilton Depression Rating Scale in unipolar depressed outpatients. *Journal of Affective Disorders*, *68*, 41–47.

Pandey, J., Verbalis, A., Robins, D. L., Boorstein, H., Klin, A., Babitz, T., ... Fein, D. (2008). Screening for autism in older and younger toddlers with the Modified Checklist for Autism in Toddlers. *Autism*, *12*, 513–535. doi: 10.1177/1362361308094503

Parker, A. J. R., Marshall, E. J., & Ball, D. M. (2008). Diagnosis and management of alcohol use disorders. *British Medical Journal, 336*, 496–501. doi: 10.1136/bmj.39483.457708.80

Parker, S. C., Lyons, J., & Bonner, J. (2005). Eating disorders in graduate students: Exploring the SCOFF questionnaire as a simple screening tool. *Journal of American College Health, 54*, 103–107.

Pastor, P. N., & Reuben, C. A. (2008). Diagnosed attention deficit hyperactivity disorder and learning disability: United States, 2004–2006. National Center for Health Statistics. *Vital Health Statistics, 10*(237), 1–14.

Perry, L., Morgan, J., Reid, F., Brunton, J., O'Brien, A., Luck, A., & Lacey, H. (2002). Screening for symptoms of eating disorders: Reliability of the SCOFF screening tool with written compared to oral delivery. *International Journal of Eating Disorders, 32*, 466–472. doi: 10.1002/eat.10093

Pitanupong, J., Liabsuetrakul, T., & Vittayanont, A. (2007). Validation of the Thai Edinburgh Postnatal Depression Scale for screening postpartum depression. *Psychiatry Research, 149*, 253–259.

Ponniah, K., & Hollon, S. D. (2009). Empirically supported psychological treatments for adult acute stress disorder and posttraumatic stress disorder: A review. *Depression and Anxiety, 26*, 1086–1109. doi: 10.1002/da.20635

Posserud, M.-B., Lundervold, A. J., & Gillberg, C. (2006). Autistic features in a total population of 7–9 year-old children assessed by the ASSQ (Autism Spectrum Screening Questionnaire). *Journal of Child Psychology and Psychiatry, 47*, 167–175. doi: 10.1111/j.1469-7610.2005.01462.x

Posserud, M.-B., Lundervold, A. J., & Gillberg, C. (2009). Validation of the Autism Spectrum Screening Questionnaire in a total population sample. *Journal of Autism & Developmental Disorders, 39*, 126–134. doi: 10.1007/s10803-008-0609-z

Posserud, M.-B., Lundervold, A. J., Steijnen, M. C., Verhoeven, S., Stormark, K. M., & Gillberg, C. (2008). Factor analysis of the Autism Spectrum Screening Questionnaire. *Autism, 12*, 99–112. doi: 10.1177/1362361307085268

Powers, M. B., Gillihan, S. J., Rosenfield, D., Jerud, A. B., & Foa, E. B. (2012). Reliability and validity of the PDS and PSS-I among participants with PTSD and alcohol dependence. *Journal of Anxiety Disorders, 26*, 617–623. doi: 10.1016/j.janxdis.2012.02.013

Prigerson, H. G., Ahmed, I., Silverman, G. K., Saxena, A. K., Maciejewski, P. K., Jacobs, S. C., ... Hamirani, M. (2002). Rates and risks of complicated grief among psychiatric clinic patients in Karachi, Pakistan. *Death Studies, 26*, 781–792. doi: 10.1080/074811802 90106571

Prigerson, H. G., & Jacobs, S. (2001). Traumatic grief as a distinct disorder: A rational, consensus criteria, and a preliminary empirical test. In M. S. Stroebe, R. O. Hansson, W. Stroebe, & H. Schut (Eds.), *Handbook of bereavement research: Consequences, coping, and care* (pp. 613–637). Washington, DC: American Psychological Association.

Prigerson, H. G., Maciejewski, P. K., Reynolds, III, C. F., Bierhals, A. J., Newsom, J. T., Fasiczka, A., ... Miller, M. (1995). Inventory of Complicated Grief: A scale to measure maladaptive symptoms of loss. *Psychiatry Research, 59*, 65–79.

Prigerson, H. G., Shear, M. K., Jacobs, S. C., Reynolds, III, C. F., Maciejewski, P. J., Davidson, J. R. T., ... Zisook, S. (1999). Consensus criteria for traumatic grief: A preliminary empirical test. *The British Journal of Psychiatry, 174*, 67–73. doi: 10.1192/bjp.174.1.67

Pulay, A. J., Stinson, F. S., Dawson, D. A., Goldstein, R. B., Chou, S. P., Huang, B., ... Grant, B. F. (2009). Prevalence, correlates, disability, and comorbidity of DSM-IV schizotypal personality disorder: Results from the wave 2 National Epidemiologic Survey on Alcohol and Related Conditions. *The Primary Care Companion to the Journal of Clinical Psychiatry*, *11*, 53–67.

Radloff, L. S. (1977). The CES-D scale: A self-report depression scale for research in the general population. *Applied Psychological Measurement*, *1*, 385–401.

Ramos-Quiroga J. A., Daigre, C., Valero, S., Bosch, R., Gómez-Barros, N., Nogueira, M., ... Casas, M. (2009). Validation of the Spanish version of the Attention Deficit Hyperactivity Disorder Adult Screening Scale (ASRS v. 1.1): A novel scoring strategy. *Reviews Neurology*, *48*, 449–452.

Raven, M., Stuart, G. W., & Jureidini, J. (2012). "Prodromal" diagnosis of psychosis: Ethical problems in research and clinical practice. *Australian & New Zealand Journal of Psychiatry*, *46*, 64–65. doi: 10.1177/0004867411428917

Rehm, L. P., & O'Hara, M. W. (1985). Item characteristics of the Hamilton Rating Scale for Depression. *Journal of Psychiatric Research*, *19*, 31–41.

Reighard, F. T., & Evans, M. L. (1995). Use of the Edinburgh Postnatal Depression Scale in a southern, rural population in the United States. *Progress in Neuro-Psychopharmacology and Biological Psychiatry*, *19*, 1219–1224. doi: 10.1016/0278-5846 (95)00238-3

Reijonen, J. H., Pratt, H. D., Patel, D. R., & Greydanus, D. E. (2003). Eating disorders in the adolescent population: An overview. *Journal of Adolescent Research*, *18*, 209–222. doi: 10.1177/0743558403018003002

Rist, F., Glöckner-Rist, A., & Demmel, R. (2009). The Alcohol Use Disorders Identification Test revisited: Establishing its structure using nonlinear factor analysis and identifying subgroups of respondents using latent class factor analysis. *Drug and Alcohol Dependence*, *100*, 71–82. doi: 10.1016/j.drugalcdep.2008.09.008

Rivet, T. T., & Matson, J. L. (2011). Review of gender differences in core symptomatology in autism spectrum disorders. *Research in Autism Spectrum Disorders*, *5*, 957–976. doi: 10.1016/j.rasd.2010.12.003

Roberts, N. P., Kitchiner, N. J., Kenardy, J., & Bisson, J. I. (2009). Systematic review and meta-analysis of multiple-session early interventions following traumatic events. *The American Journal of Psychiatry*, *166*, 293–301. doi: 10.1176/appi.ajp.2008.08040590

Robins, D. L., Fein, D., Barton, M. L., & Green, J. A. (2001). The Modified Checklist for Autism in Toddlers: An initial study investigating the early detection of autism and pervasive developmental disorders. *Journal of Autism and Developmental Disorders*, *31*, 131–144.

Rolfsnes, E. S., & Idsoe, T. (2011). School-based intervention programs for PTSD symptoms: A review and meta-analysis. *Journal of Traumatic Stress*, *24*, 155–165. doi: 10.1002/jts.20622

Romera, I., Pérez, V., Menchón, J. M., Polavieja, P., & Gilaberte, I. (2011). Optimal cutoff point of the Hamilton Rating Scale for Depression according to normal levels of social and occupational functioning. *Psychiatry Research*, *186*, 133–137.

Rosen, J. C., Jones, A., Ramirez, E., & Waxman, S. (1996). Body Shape Questionnaire: Studies of validity and reliability. *International Journal of Eating Disorders, 20*, 315–319.

Rosen, J. L. Miller, T. J., D'Andrea, J. T., McGlashan, T. H., & Woods, S. W. (2006). Comorbid diagnoses in patients meeting criteria for the schizophrenia prodrome. *Schizophrenia Research, 85*, 124–131. doi: 10.1016/j.schres.2006.03.034

Rosenberg, R. E., Kaufmann, W. E., Law, J. K., & Law, P. A. (2011). Parent report of community psychiatric comorbid diagnoses in autism spectrum disorders. *Autism Research & Treatment, 2011*, 1–10. doi: 10.1155/2011/405849

Rosenman, S., & Anderson, P. (2011). Does prodromal diagnosis delay early intervention? *The Australian & New Zealand Journal of Psychiatry, 45*, 509–514. doi: 10.3109/00048674.2011.566549

Rossini, E. D., & O'Connor, M. A. (1995). Retrospective self-reported symptoms of attention-deficit hyperactivity disorder: Reliability of the Wender Utah Rating Scale. *Psychological Reports, 77*, 751–754.

Rousseau, A., Knotter, A., Barbe, P., Raich, R. M., & Chabrol, H. (2005). Validation of the French version of the Body Shape Questionnaire. *L'Encéphale: Revue de Psychiatrie Clinique Biologique et Thérapeutique, 31*, 162–173.

Ruggiero, K. J., Del Ben, K., Scotti, J. R., & Rabalais, A. E. (2003). Psychometric properties of the PTSD Checklist—Civilian version. *Journal of Traumatic Stress, 16*, 495–502. doi: 10.1023/A:1025714729117

Ruiz, M. A., Zamorano, E., García-Campayo, J., Pardo, A., Freire, O., & Rejas, J. (2011). Validity of the GAD-7 scale as an outcome measure of disability in patients with generalized anxiety disorders in primary care. *Journal of Affective Disorders, 128*, 277–286.

Ruta, L., Mazzone, D., Mazzone, L., Wheelwright, S., & Baron-Cohen, S. (2012). The Autism-Spectrum Quotient—Italian version: A cross-cultural confirmation of the broader autism phenotype. *Journal of Autism and Developmental Disorders, 42*, 625–633.

Ryu, H. R., Lyle, R. M., Galer-Unti, R. A., & Black, D. R. (1999). Cross-cultural assessment of eating disorders: Psychometric characteristics of a Korean version of the Eating Disorder Inventory—2 and the Bulimia Test—Revised. *Eating Disorders, 7*, 109–122.

Saha, S., Chant, D., Welham, J., & McGrath, J. (2005). How prevalent is schizophrenia? *Public Library of Science Medicine, 2*, 362–363. doi: 10.1371/journal.pmed.0020146

Santis, R., Garmendia, M. L, Acuna, G., Alvarado, M. E., & Arteaga, O. (2009). The Alcohol Use Disorders Identification Test (AUDIT) as a screening instrument for adolescents. *Drug and Alcohol Dependence, 103*, 155–158. doi: 10.1016/j.drugalcdep.2009.01.017

Santor, D. A., Zuroff, D. C., Ramsay, J. O., Cervantes, P., & Palacios, J. (1995). Examining scale discriminability in the BDI and CES-D as a function of depressive severity. *Psychological Assessment, 7*, 131–139. doi: 10.1037/1040-3590.7.2.131

Saracino, J., Noseworthy, J., Steiman, M., Reisinger, L, & Fombonne, E. (2010). Diagnostic and assessment issues in autism surveillance and prevalence. *Journal of Developmental & Physical Disabilities, 22*, 317–330. doi: 10.1007/s10882-010-9205-1

Sarin, F., Wallin, L, & Widerlööv, B. (2011). Cognitive behavior therapy for schizophrenia: A meta-analytical review of randomized controlled trials. *Nordic Journal of Psychiatry, 65*, 162–174. doi: 10.3109/08039488.2011.577188

Saunders, J. B., Aasland, O. G., Babor, T. F., De La Fuente, J. R., & Grant, M. (1993). Development of the alcohol use disorders identification test (AUDIT): WHO collaborative project on early detection of persons with harmful alcohol consumption II. *Addiction, 88*, 791–803.

Schinka, J. A., Brown, L. M., Borenstein, A. R., & Mortimer, J. A. (2007). Confirmatory factor analysis of the PTSD Checklist in the elderly. *Journal of Traumatic Stress, 20*, 281–289. doi: 10.1002/jts.20202

Schmidt, A., & Barry, K. L. (1995). Detection of problem drinkers: The Alcohol Use Disorders Identification Test (AUDIT). *Southern Medical Journal, 88*, 52–59.

Schneier, F. R., Foose, T. E., Hasin, D. S., Heimberg, R. G., Liu, S.-M., Grant, B. F., & Blanco, C. (2010). Social anxiety disorder and alcohol use disorder co-morbidity in the National Epidemiologic Survey on alcohol and related conditions. *Psychological Medicine: A Journal of Research in Psychiatry and the Allied Sciences, 40*, 977–988. doi: 10.1017/S0033291709991231

Selin, K. H. (2003). Test-retest reliability of the Alcohol Use Disorders Identification Test in a general population sample. *Alcoholism: Clinical and Experimental Research, 27*, 1428–1435.

Shearin, E. N., Russ, M. J., Hull, J. W., Clarkin, J. F., & Smith, G. P. (1994). Construct validity of the Three-Factor Eating Questionnaire: Flexible and rigid control subscales. *International Journal of Eating Disorders, 16*, 187–198.

Shelby, R. A., Golden-Kreutz, D. M., & Andersen, B. L. (2005). Mismatch of posttraumatic stress disorder (PTSD) symptoms and DSM-IV symptom clusters in a cancer sample: Exploratory factor analysis of the PTSD Checklist—Civilian version. *Journal of Traumatic Stress, 18*, 347–357. doi: 10.1002/jts.20033

Shields, A. L., Guttmannova, K., & Caruso, J. C. (2004). An examination of the factor structure of the Alcohol Use Disorders Identification Test in two high-risk samples. *Substance Use & Misuse, 39*, 1161–1182. doi: 10.1081/JA-120038034

Simmons, M. B., & Hetrick, S. E. (2012). "Prodromal" research and clinical services: The imperative for shared decision-making. *The Australian & New Zealand Journal of Psychiatry, 46*, 66. doi: 10.1177/0004867411427813

Sin, G.-L., Abdin, E., & Lee, J. (2012). The PSS-SR as a screening tool for PTSD in first-episode psychosis patients. *Early Intervention in Psychiatry, 6*, 191–194. doi: 10.1111/j.1751-7893.2011.00327.x

Singh, S. P., & Singh, V. (2009). Meta-analysis of the efficacy of adjunctive NMDA receptor modulators in chronic schizophrenia. *CNS Drugs, 25*, 859–885.

Smith, M. C., & Thelen, M. H. (1984). Development and validation of a test for bulimia. *Journal of Consulting and Clinical Psychology, 52*, 863–872.

Snow, A. V., & Lecavalier, L. (2008). Sensitivity and specificity of the Modified Checklist for Autism in Toddlers and the Social Communication Questionnaire in preschoolers suspected of having pervasive developmental disorders. *Autism, 12*, 627–645. doi: 10.1177/1362361308097116

Spear, S., Tillman, S., Moss, C., Gong-Guy, E., Ransom, L., & Rawson, R. A. (2009). Another way of talking about substance abuse: Substance abuse screening and brief intervention in a mental health clinic. *Journal of Human Behavior in the Social Environment, 19*, 959–977. doi: 10.1080/10911350902992797

Spence, S. H. (1997). Structure of anxiety symptoms among children: A confirmatory factor-analytic study. *Journal of Abnormal Psychology, 106*, 280–297.

Spence, S. H. (1998). A measure of anxiety symptoms among children. *Behaviour Research and Therapy, 36*, 545–566.

Spence, S. H., Barrett, P. M., & Turner, C. M. (2003). Psychometric properties of the Spence Children's Anxiety Scale with young adolescents. *Journal of Anxiety Disorders, 17*, 605–625.

Spence, S. H., Rapee, R., McDonald, C., & Ingram, M. (2001). The structure of anxiety symptoms among preschoolers. *Behaviour Research and Therapy, 39*, 1293–1316.

Spiegel, D., Koopman, C., Cardeña, E., & Classen, C. (1996). Dissociative symptoms in the diagnosis of acute stress disorder. In L. Michelson & W. J. Ray (Eds.), *Handbook of dissociation* (pp. 367–380). New York, NY: Plenum.

Spitzer, R. L., Kroenke, K., Williams, J. B., & Löwe, B. A. (2006). Brief measure for assessing generalized anxiety disorder: The GAD-7. *Archives of Internal Medicine, 166*, 1092–1097.

Steel, C., Garety, P. A., Freeman, D., Craig, E., Kuipers, E., Bebbington, P., ... Dunn, G. (2007). The multidimensional measurement of the positive symptoms of psychosis. *International Journal of Methods in Psychiatric Research, 16*, 88–96. doi: 10.1002/mpr.203

Stein, M. A., Sandoval, R., Szumowski, E., Roizen, N., Reinecke, M. A., Blondis, T. A., & Klein, Z. (1995). Psychometric characteristics of the Wender Utah Rating Scale (WURS): Reliability and factor structure for men and women. *Psychopharmacology Bulletin, 31*, 425–433.

Stein, M. B., McQuaid, J. R., Pedrelli, P., Lenox, R., & McCahill, M. E. (2000). Posttraumatic stress disorder in the primary care medical setting. *General Hospital Psychiatry, 22*, 261–269. doi: 10.1016/S0163-8343(00)00080-3

Stewart, M. E., & Austin, E. J. (2009). The structure of the Autism-Spectrum Quotient (AQ): Evidence from a student sample in Scotland. *Personality and Individual Differences, 47*, 224–228. doi: 10.1016/j.paid.2009.03.004

Stice, E., Fisher, M., & Martinez, E. (2004). Eating Disorder Diagnostic Scale: Additional evidence of reliability and validity. *Psychological Assessment, 16*, 60–71. doi: 10.1037/1040-3590.16.1.60

Stice, E., Telch, C. F., & Rizvi, S. L. (2000). Development and validation of the Eating Disorder Diagnostic Scale: A brief self-report measure of anorexia, bulimia, and binge-eating disorder. *Psychological Assessment, 12*, 123–131. doi: 10.1037//1040-3590.12.2.123

Stinson, F. S., Grant, B. F., Dawson, D. A., Ruan, W. J., Huang, B., & Saha, T. (2006). Comorbidity between DSM-IV alcohol and specific drug use disorders in the United States: Results from the National Epidemiologic Survey on Alcohol and Related Conditions. *Alcohol Research & Health, 29*, 94–106.

Stommel, M., Given, B. A., Given, C. W., Kalaian, H. A., Schulz, R., & McCorkle, R. (1993). Gender bias in the measurement properties of the Center for Epidemiologic Studies–Depression Scale (CES-D). *Psychiatry Research, 49*, 239–250.

Storch, E. A., Murphy, T. K., Adkins, J. W., Lewin, A. B., Geffken, G. R., Johns, N. B., ... Goodman, W. K. (2006). The Children's Yale-Brown Obsessive-Compulsive Scale:

Psychometric properties of child- and parent-report formats. *Journal of Anxiety Disorders, 20*, 1055–1070.

Storch, E. A., Murphy, T. K., Geffken, G. R., Soto, O., Sajid, M., Allen, P...Goodman, W. K. (2004). Psychometric evaluation of the Children's Yale-Brown Obsessive-Compulsive Scale. *Psychiatry Research, 129*, 91–98.

Strine, T. W., Lesesne, C. A., Okoro, C. A., McGuire, L. C., Chapman, D. P., Balluz, L. S., & Mokdad, A. H. (2006). Emotional and behavioral difficulties and impairments in everyday functioning among children with a history of attention-deficit/hyperactivity disorder. *Preventing Chronic Disease, 3*(2), A52.

Stunkard, A. J., & Messick, S. (1985). The Three-Factor Eating Questionnaire to measure dietary restraint, disinhibition, and hunger. *Journal of Psychosomatic Research, 29*, 71–83.

Su, K. P., Chiu, T. H., Huang, C. L., Ho, M., Lee, C. C. Wu, P. L., ... Pariante, C. M. (2007). Different cutoff points for different trimesters? The use of Edinburgh Postnatal Depression Scale and Beck Depression Inventory to screen for depression in pregnant Taiwanese women. *General Hospital Psychiatry, 29*, 436–441. doi: 10.1016/j.genhosp psych.2007.05.005

Subramaniam, M., Cheok, C., Verma, S., Wong, J., & Chong, S. A. (2010). Validity of a brief screening instrument: CRAFFT in a multiethnic Asian population. *Addictive Behaviors, 35*, 1102–1104. doi: 10.1016/j.addbeh.2010.08.004

Swanson, S. A., Crow, S. J., Le Grange, D., Swendsen, J., & Merikangas, K. R. (2011). Prevalence and correlates of eating disorders in adolescents: Results from the national comorbidity survey replication adolescent supplement. *Archives of General Psychiatry, 68*, 714–723. doi: 10.1001/archgenpsychiatry.2011.22

Thelen, M. H., Farmer, J., Wonderlich, S., & Smith, M. (1991). A revision of the bulimia test: The BULIT-R. *Psychological Assessment, 3*, 119–124.

Thelen, M. H., Mintz, L. B., & Vander Wal, J. S. (1996). The Bulimia Test—Revised: Validation with DSM-IV criteria for bulimia nervosa. *Psychological Assessment, 8*, 219–221.

Tholin, S., Rasmussen, F., Tynelius, P., & Karlsson, J. (2005). Genetic and environmental influences on eating behavior: The Swedish Young Male Twins Study. *American Journal of Clinical Nutrition, 81*, 564–569.

Thurber, S., Snow, M., & Honts, C. R. (2002). The Zung Self-Rating Depression Scale: Convergent validity and diagnostic discrimination. *Assessment, 9*, 401–405.

Timko, C., Moos, R. H., Finney, J. W., & Lesar, M. D. (2000). Long-term outcomes of alcohol use disorders: Comparing untreated individuals with those in alcoholics anonymous and formal treatment. *Journal of Studies on Alcohol, 61*, 529–540.

Timmerman, G. M. (1999). Binge Eating Scale. Further assessment of validity and reliability. *Journal of Applied Biobehavioral Research, 4*, 1–12. doi: 10.1111/j.1751-9861. 1999.tb00051.x

Tolin, D. F., & Foa, E. B. (2008). Sex differences in trauma and posttraumatic stress disorder: A quantitative review of 25 years of research. *Psychological Trauma: Theory, Research, Practice, and Policy, S*, 37–85. doi: 10.1037/1942-9681.S.1.37

Tolin, D. F., Frost, R. O., & Steketee, G. (2010). A brief interview for assessing compulsive hoarding: The Hoarding Rating Scale-Interview. *Psychiatry Research, 178*, 147–152. doi: 10.1016/j.psychres.2009.05.001

Trajković, G., Starčević, V., Latas, M., Leštarević, M., Ille, T., Bukumirić, Z., & Marinković, J. (2011). Reliability of the Hamilton Rating Scale for Depression: A meta-analysis over a period of 49 years. *Psychiatry Research, 189*, 1–9.

Trickey, D., Siddaway, A. P., Meiser-Stedman, R., Serpell, L., & Field, A. P. (2012). A meta-analysis of risk factors of post-traumatic stress disorder in children and adolescents. *Clinical Psychology Review, 32*, 122–138. doi: 10.1016/j.cpr.2011.12.001

Van Dam, N. T., & Earleywine, M. (2011). Validation of the Center for Epidemiologic Studies Depression Scale—Revised (CES-D-R): Pragmatic depression assessment in the general population. *Psychiatry Research, 186*, 128–132.

Ventola, P., Kleinman, J., Pandey, J., Wilson, L., Esser, E., Boorstein, H., ... Fein, D. (2007). Differentiating between autism spectrum disorders and other developmental disabilities in children who failed a screening instrument for ASD. *Journal of Autism & Developmental Disorders, 37*, 425–436. doi: 10.1007/s10803-006-0177-z

Volk, R. J., Steinbauer, J. R., Cantor, S. B., & Holzer, C. E. (1997). The Alcohol Use Disorders Identification Test (AUDIT) as a screen for at-risk drinking in primary care patients of different racial/ethnic backgrounds. *Addition, 92*, 197–206.

von der Pahlen, B., Santtila, P., Witting, K., Varjonen, M., Jern, P., Johansson, A., & Sandnabba, N. K. (2008). Factor structure of the Alcohol Use Disorders Identification Test (AUDIT) for men and women in different age groups. *Journal of Studies on Alcohol and Drugs, 69*, 616–621.

Wade, T. D., Bergin, J. L., Tiggemann, M., Bulik, C. M., & Fairburn, C. G. (2006). Prevalence and long-term course of lifetime eating disorders in an adult Australian twin cohort. *Australian and New Zealand Journal of Psychiatry, 40*, 121–128. doi: 10.1111/j.1440-1614.2006.01758.x

Waelde, L. C., Koopman, C., Rierdan, J., & Spiegel, D. (2001). Symptoms of acute stress disorder and posttraumatic stress disorder following exposure to disastrous flooding. *Journal of Trauma & Dissociation, 2*, 37–52. doi: 10.1300/J229v02n02_04

Wakabayashi, A., Baron-Cohen, S., Uchiyama, T., Yoshida, Y., Tojo, Y., Kuroda, M., & Wheelwright, S. (2007). The Autism-Spectrum Quotient (AQ) Children's version in Japan: A cross-cultural comparison. *Journal of Autism and Developmental Disorders, 37*, 491–500. doi: 10.1007/s10803-006-0181-3

Wakabayashi, A., Baron-Cohen, S., Wheelwright, S., & Tojo, Y. (2006). The Autism-Spectrum Quotient (AQ) in Japan: A cross-cultural comparison. *Journal of Autism and Developmental Disorders, 36*, 263–270. doi: 10.1007/s10803-005-0061-2

Wakabayashi, A., Tojo, Y., Baron-Cohen, S., & Wheelwright, S. (2004). The Autism-Spectrum Quotient (AQ) Japanese version: Evidence from high-functioning clinical group and normal adults. *Japanese Journal of Psychology, 75*, 78–84. doi: 10.4992/jjpsy.75.78

Walker, E. A., Newman, E., Dobie, D. J., Ciechanowski, P., & Katon, W. (2002). Validation of the PTSD Checklist in an HMO sample of women. *General Hospital Psychiatry, 24*, 375–380. doi: 10.1016/S0163-8343(02)00203-7

Wang, L., Li, Z., Shi, Z., Zhang, Y., & Shen, J. (2010). Factor structure of acute stress disorder symptoms in Chinese earthquake victims: A confirmatory factor analysis of the Acute Stress Disorder Scale. *Personality and Individual Differences, 48*, 798–802. doi: 10.1016/j.paid.2010.01.027

Wang, M.-C., Dai, X.-Y., & Wan, J. (2009). Factor structure of PTSD Checklist: A confirmatory factor analysis study in adolescents from earthquake region. *Chinese Journal of Clinical Psychology, 17*, 420–423.

Wang, P. S., Lane, M., Olfson, M., Pincus, H. A., Wells, K. B., & Kessler, R. C. (2005). Twelve month use of mental health services in the United States. *Archives of General Psychiatry, 62*, 629–640.

Weathers, F. W., Litz, B. T., Herman, D. W., Huska, J. A., & Keane, T. M. (1993). The PTSD Checklist (PCL): Reliability, validity, and diagnostic utility. Paper presented at the Annual Meeting of the International Society for Traumatic Stress Studies, San Antonio, TX, October.

Weinstein, A., & Lejoyeux, M. (2010). Internet addiction or excessive Internet use. *The American Journal of Drug and Alcohol Abuse, 36*, 277–283. doi: 10.3109/00952990.2010.491880

Werrett, J., & Clifford, C. (2006). Validation of the Punjabi version of the Edinburgh postnatal depression scale (EPDS). *International Journal of Nursing Studies, 43*, 227–236.

Wierzbicki, M. (2005). Reliability and validity of the Wender Utah Rating Scale for college students. *Psychological Reports, 96*, 833–839. doi: 10.2466/pr0.96.3.833-839

Wilkins, K. C., Lang, A. J., & Norman, S. B. (2011). Synthesis of the psychometric properties of the PTSD checklist (PCL) military, civilian, and specific versions. *Depression and Anxiety, 28*, 596–606. doi: 10.1002/da.20837

Wilkinson, A. (2010). School-age children with autism spectrum disorders: Screening and identification. *European Journal of Special Needs Education, 25*, 211–223. doi: 10.1080/08856257.2010.492928

Williams, J. B. (1988). A structured interview guide for the Hamilton Depression Rating Scale. *Archives of General Psychiatry, 45*, 742–747.

Williams, J. L., Monahan, C. J., & McDevitt-Murphy, M. E. (2011). Factor structure of the PTSD Checklist in a sample of OEF/OIF veterans presenting to primary care: Specific and nonspecific aspects of dysphoria. *Journal of Psychopathology and Behavioral Assessment, 33*, 514–522. doi: 10.1007/s10862-011-9248-3

Wohlfarth, T. D., van den Brink, W., Winkel, F. W., & ter Smitten, M. (2003). Screening for posttraumatic stress disorder: An evaluation of two self-report scales among crime victims. *Psychological Assessment, 15*, 101–109. doi: 10.1037/1040-3590.15.1.101

Wolraich, M. L., Feurer, I. D., Hannah, J. N., Baumgaertel, A., & Pinnock, T. Y. (1998). Obtaining systematic teacher reports of disruptive behavior disorders utilizing DSM-IV. *Journal of Abnormal Child Psychology, 26*(2), 141–152.

Wolraich, M. L., Lambert, W., Doffing, M. A., Bickman, L., Simmons, T., & Worley, K. (2003). Psychometric properties of the Vanderbilt AD/HD Diagnostic Parent Rating Scale in a referred population. *Journal of Pediatric Psychology, 28*, 559–568. doi: 10.1093/jpepsy/jsg046

Woodbury-Smith, M. R., Robinson, J., Wheelwright, S., & Baron-Cohen, S. (2005). Screening adults for Asperger syndrome using the AQ: A preliminary study of its diagnostic validity in clinical practice. *Journal of Autism and Developmental Disorders, 35*, 331–335. doi: 10.1007/s10803-005-3300-7

World Health Organization. (2012). *Schizophrenia*. Retrieved from http://www.who.int/mental_health/management/schizophrenia/en/

Wouters, S. G. M., & Spek, A. A. (2011). The use of the Autism-spectrum Quotient in differentiating high-functioning adults with autism, adults with schizophrenia and a neurotypical adult control group. *Research in Autism Spectrum Disorders, 5*, 1169–1175. doi: 10.1016/j.rasd.2011.01.002

Wright, K., & Poulin-Dubois, D. (2012). Modified Checklist for Autism in Toddlers (M-CHAT) screening at 18 months of age predicts concurrent understanding of desires, word learning and expressive vocabulary. *Research in Autism Spectrum Disorders, 6*, 184–192. doi: 10.1016/j.rasd.2011.04.004

Yama, B., Freeman, T., Graves, E., Yuan, S., & Campbell, M. K. (2012). Examination of the properties of the Modified Checklist for Autism in Toddlers (M-CHAT) in a population sample. *Journal of Autism and Developmental Disorders, 42*, 23–34. doi: 10.1007/s10803-011-1211-3

Yang, F. M., & Jones, R. N. (2007). Center for Epidemiologic Studies–Depression scale (CES-D) item response bias found with Mantel-Haenszel method was successfully replicated using latent variable modeling. *Journal of Clinical Epidemiology, 60*(11), 1195–1200.

Yeh, C. B., Gau, S. S., Kessler, R. C., & Wu, Y. Y. (2008). Psychometric properties of the Chinese version of the adult AD/HD Self-report Scale. *International Journal of Methods Psychiatry Research, 17*(1), 45–54.

Yung, A. R. (2012). Early intervention in psychosis: Evidence, evidence gaps, criticism, and confusion. *Australian & New Zealand Journal of Psychiatry, 46*, 7–9. doi: 10.1177/0004867411432205

Yung, A. R., Nelson, B., Thompson, A., & Wood, S. J. (2010). The psychosis threshold in ultra high risk (prodromal) research: Is it valid? *Schizophrenia Research, 120*, 1–6. doi: 10.1016/j.schres.2010.03.014

Zaroff, C., & Uhm, S. (2012). Prevalence of autism spectrum disorders and influence of country of measurement and ethnicity. *Social Psychiatry & Psychiatric Epidemiology, 47*, 395–398. doi: 10.1007/s00127-011-0350-3

Zheng, Y. P., Zhao, J. P., Phillips, M., Liu, J. B., Cai, M. F., Sun, S. Q., & Huang, M. F. (1988). Validity and reliability of the Chinese Hamilton Depression Rating Scale. *British Journal of Psychiatry, 152*, 660–664.

Zisook, S., Simon, N. M., Reynolds, C. F. III, Pies, R., Lebowitz, B., Young, I. T., ... Shear, M. K. (2010). Bereavement, complicated grief, and DSM, part 2: Complicated grief. *Journal of Clinical Psychiatry, 71*, 1097–1098. doi: 10.4088/JCP.10ac06391blu

Zung, W. K., Richards, C. B., & Short, M. J. (1965). Self-Rating Depression Scale in an outpatient clinic: Further validation of the SDS. *Archives of General Psychiatry, 13*, 508–515.

Index

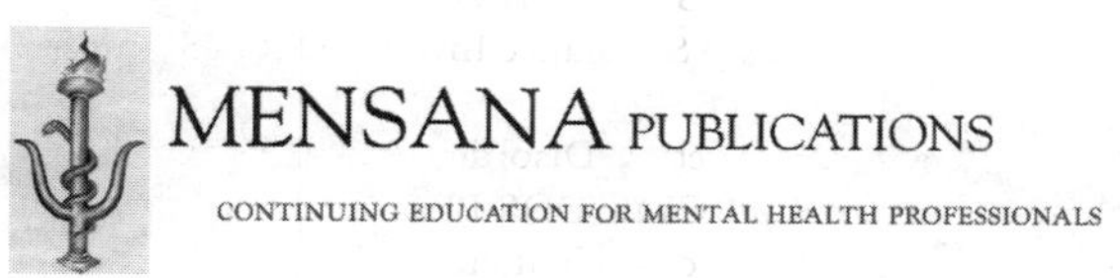

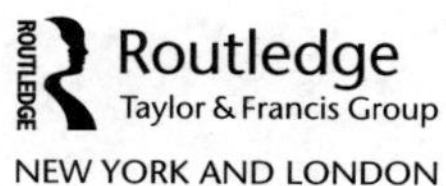

NEW YORK AND LONDON

An accredited continuing education component has been developed for this book by the author in partnership with Routledge and Mensana Publications. The CE offer is worth 6 hours of continuing education credit and may be purchased from the website below:

www.mensanapublications.com